T0185487

Chinese Medicine Periodicals from the Late Qing and Republican China:
An Overview

Chinese Medicine Periodicals from the Late Qing and Republican China: An Overview

Edited by

Duan Yishan

Translated by

Stephen Boyanton

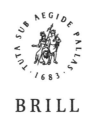

BRILL

LEIDEN | BOSTON

This book is a result of the translation license agreement between Shanghai Lexicographical Publishing House and Koninklijke Brill NV. This book includes English translations of part of the Chinese book, entitled *Compilation of Chinese Medicine Periodicals from the Late Qing and Republican Periods: An Abstracted Table of Contents*《中国近代中医药期刊汇编总目提要》(*Zhongguo jindai zhongyiyao qikan huibian zongmu tiyao*) with financial support from Shanghai Translation and Publication Fund (上海翻译出版促进计划).

Library of Congress Cataloging-in-Publication Data

Names: Duan, Yishan, editor. | Boyanton, Stephen, translator.
Title: Chinese medicine periodicals from the late Ging and Republican China: an overview / edited by Duan Yishan ; translated by Stephen Boyanton.
Other titles: Chinese medical periodicals from the late Ging and Republican China
Description: English edition. | Leiden ; Boston : Brill, 2020. | English edition, 2020. Copyrighted 2012 by Shanghai Lexicographical Publishing House. | In English. Periodical titles in both English and Chinese.
Identifiers: LCCN 2019044692 | ISBN 9789004420724 (paperback)
Subjects: LCSH: Medicine, Chinese—Periodicals—History. | Medicine, Chinese—Periodicals—Bibliography. | Medicine—Periodicals—History. | Medicine—Periodicals—Bibliography. | Medicine, Chinese—History—19th century. | Medicine, Chinese—History—20th century. | Medicine—Translations into English—Bibliography.
Classification: LCC R601 .C45 2020 | DDC 610.951—dc23
LC record available at https://lccn.loc.gov/2019044692

Typeface for the Latin, Greek, and Cyrillic scripts: "Brill". See and download: brill.com/brill-typeface.

ISBN 978-90-04-42072-4 (paperback)

This book is printed on acid-free paper and produced in a sustainable manner.

Contents

Introduction

In 2012, Shanghai University of Traditional Chinese Medicine and Shanghai Lexicographical Publishing House jointly published the *Compilation of Chinese Medicine Periodicals from the Late Qing and Republican Periods*, in print. The *Compilation*, a collection of 49 periodicals on Chinese medicine published in the late Qing and Republican periods in China, includes 212 books in 5 parts of more than 120,000 pages.

This collection includes published documents authored by prominent figures both in support of, and opposed to, Chinese medicine. The periodicals included in this collection are among the oldest, most influential and authoritative of all scholarship on Chinese medicine from the late Qing and Republican periods. The late Qing and Republican eras are crucial periods to the development of medicine and science in China. Considered one of the best sources for observing the changing nature of medical practice and education during the late Qing and Republican eras in China, this collection provides unique insight into not only the modern transformation of Chinese medicine, but also the larger role of medicine in Chinese society. The *Compilation* is a massive primary source not only for understanding the modern transformation of Chinese medicine, but also the larger role of medicine in Chinese society. It is hoped that this *Compilation* would stimulate a multitude of new research projects.

The periodicals included are both aged and rare. The editorial team worked with over 50 libraries to compile them all together in this work. To help the collection reach a wider audience, Shanghai Lexicographical Publishing House granted Brill the exclusive rights in 2017 to develop and distribute the online version, i.e., the *Compilation of Chinese Medicine Periodicals Online, 1897–1952*. To help English readers have a better understanding of the periodicals included in this collection, Brill provided an English translation of the overview of each periodical, selected from the Chinese book, entitled *Compilation of Chinese Medicine Periodicals from the Late Qing and Republican Periods: An Abstracted Table of Contents*, edited by Duan Yishan 段逸山. The English translations of these overviews, which have been provided online at the Brill website since 2017, are now included in this booklet.

Wang Youpeng, editor at Shanghai Lexicographical Publishing House published an article (in Chinese), entitled *A Humanist Analysis on Periodicals of Chinese Medicine from the Late Qing and Republican Periods*, to explain how this product was developed and its academic significance. This article has been

translated into English by David Luesink and the English translation was published in *Twentieth-Century China*, 40, 1, 69–78, January 2015. With permission
by the author, translator and the journal publisher, the English translation of
Wang's article is included in this booklet as Appendix.

This booklet includes an English translation of the overviews 概況 of all the periodicals included in the Compilation of Chinese Medicine Periodicals from the Late Qing and Republican Periods (1897–1952). There are 49 periodicals included in the collection. There are a total of 48 overviews with each overview for one periodical, except for Overview #7 which includes two periodicals (Shanghai's *Chinese Medicine Magazine* and Shanghai's *National Medicine Magazine*).

1. Report of the Academy of Beneficial Aid (Liji xuetang bao 利濟學堂報)

On 18th day of the 12th month of the twenty-second year of the *guangxu* reign period of the Qing dynasty (January 20th, 1897), the *Report of the Academy of Beneficial Aid* was established by Chen Qiu 陳虬 in Wenzhou, Zhejiang, to be published by the Academy of Beneficial Aid. This periodical was printed approximately every half-month, being published on the first day of each of the twenty-four solar terms. Moreover, in accord with the theory, "The five circulatory phases and six qi begin with the solar term Great Coldness" (found in the first issue of the *Report of the Academy of Beneficial Aid*), the first day of Great Coldness of the *bing-shen* year [1896] was fixed as the beginning of the first year of publication, thus taking the twenty-four solar terms from Great Coldness to the following Small Coldness as one year. Moreover, they followed the method of calculating the five circulatory phases used in chapter seventy of the *Basic Questions* (*Suwen* 素問), "Great Discourse on the Decrees of the Five Constants," according to which the *ding-you* year [1897] is a "year of accumulated harmony." Relying on this principle, the date on the front cover of the initial issue was marked as "*Guangxu* year 23, *ding-you*," "Great Coldness of the year of accumulated harmony." For this periodical, each issue was a single volume. Each issue was approximately fifty pages. Seventeen issues are extant. No original editions have been seen for issues after the seventeenth, and several issues were published that are unknown. Shanghai Lexicographical Publishing House used the copies collected by the Wenzhou Library to compile the unpublished material of the first seventeen issues. They have been edited following the style and sequence of the original publication to produce the *Supplement to the Report of the Academy of Beneficial Aid.*

The editor-in-chief, Chen Qiu's (1851–1904), was originally named Guozhen 國珍. His courtesy name was Qingsong 慶宋, and his sobriquet was Zishan 子珊. Later on he changed his courtesy name to Zhisan 志三 and his sobriquet to Zhelu 蟄盧. He was also called Gaolaozi 皋牢子. He was from Duan'an, Zhejiang. His ancestral home was Leqing, Zhejiang. In the *ji-chou* year of the *guangxu* reign period [1889] he passed the provincial level of the imperial examination. His family was poor. From childhood, he was diligent and loved studying, and through self-study, he made something of himself. Prior to the reforms of the *wu-xu* year [1898], he and Tang Shouqian 湯壽潛 (courtesy name Zhexian 蟄仙) were called "the two Zhe 蟄 of eastern Zhejiang." Furthermore he, along with Chen Fuchen 陳黻宸 and Song Shu 宋恕—together known as

© KONINKLIJKE BRILL NV, LEIDEN, 2020 | DOI:10.1163/9789004420724_002

"the three luminaries of eastern Ou"[1]—supported the Hundred Days Reform. Chen Qiu was not only one of our countries modern reformist thinkers, he was also an eminent Chinese medicine teacher of great attainments.

In the tenth year of the *guangxu* reign period, Mr. Chen wrote *On Hospitals* (*Yiyuan yi* 醫院議), putting forth plans for the establishment of Chinese medicine hospitals and schools. The following year, he, Chen Fuchen, and He Diqi 何迪啓 pooled their resources to establish the Beneficial Aid Hospital in Wenzhou. The same year, they also established the Beneficial Aid Branch Hospital and Medical Academy in Wenzhou, thus establishing the earliest new-style Chinese medicine school. On the first day of the seventh month of the twenty-second year of the *guangxu* reign period, Huang Zunxian 黃遵憲, Wang Kangnian 汪康年, and Liang Qichao 梁啓超 founded the *Journal of Current Affairs* and set up their regional distribution office at the Beneficial Aid Hospital. Chen Qiu, while enthusiastically marketing the *Journal of Current Affairs*, also conceived the idea publishing a journal himself. After a period of preparation, he founded our country's first school journal, the *Report of the Academy of Beneficial Aid*.

Regarding the date and cause of the cessation of publication of the *Report of the Academy of Beneficial Aid*, there are historians of journalism who think that "in the wake of the failure of the Hundred Days Reform, the Qing court issued a warrant for the arrest of Chen Qiu, and the Academy of Beneficial Aid was abandoned. This journal as well then ceased publication" (Fang Hanqi 方漢奇 ed., *A History of the Journalism Profession in China* [*Zhongguo xinwen shiye shi* 中國新聞事業史], volume 1, Chinese People's University Press, 1992, p. 629). However, according to Chen Yushen's 陳玉申 research, the *Record of the Academy of Benevolent Aid*, stopped publication because it accumulated excessive losses ("Investigations into the *Report of the Academy of Benevolent Aid* [*Liji tang bao kaobian* 利濟堂報考辯]," *The Press* [*Xinwenjie* 新聞界], 2007, issue 5, p. 165). Chen further argues that if the journal ceased publication one year after its inception, during the Hundred Days Reform, the later ten plus issues should not have been completely lost. Examining the contents of the *Supplement*, it can be seen that the "Literary Records" section records a total of nine pieces of literature. In the *Records of the Academy of Benevolent Aid*, each issue usually contains three pieces of literature. We can infer that this periodical probably published three more issues after the seventeenth, for a total of twenty issues. It probably ceased publication in November of 1897.

---

1 I.e., Wenzhou.

2. Medical News (Yixue bao 醫學報)

In the fourth month of the thirtieth year of the *guangxu* reign period of the Qing dynasty (1904), *Medical News* was founded by Zhou Xueqiao 周雪樵 in Shanghai. At first it was published on his behalf by a foreign newspaper publisher. Beginning with the fifty-first issue, it was published by Ancient Fragrance Pavilion Bookshop (*Guxiangge shufang* 古香閣書坊) on his behalf. Beginning with the sixty-fourth issue, he again changed publishers, and Timely Accord Book Company (*Shuzhong shuju* 時中書局) published it on his behalf. It began as a semimonthly periodical. On the first and fifteenth day each month one issue was released. In the fifth month of the first year of the *xuantong* reign period of the Qing dynasty (1909), beginning with the 109th issue, it became a ten-day periodical. In its early stages, this journal released a total of 126 issues. Later on, owing to internal disputes, the it split into two journals. The first, with Wang Wenqiao 王問樵 as chief editor, was *Medical Bulletin* (*Yixue gongbao* 醫學公報). On the twelfth day of the twelfth month of the first year of the *xuantong* reign period, it released a single issue. Afterwards, it released two issues every month. It continued the issue numbering from the previous *Medical News* up until issue number 146, when it ceased publication. The second, with Gu Mingsheng 顧鳴盛 as editor, was *Medical News* (*Yixue bao* 醫學報). It was published in the name of a branch of the Chinese Medical Association (*Zhongguo yixue hui* 中國醫學會). It also released two issues per month, but began a new series of issue numbers. Its first issue was released on the first day of the first month of the second year of the *xuantong* reign period. After the seventh issue it ceased publication.

The given name of the founder of this journal, Zhou Xueqiao (1864–1910), was 維翰, but he went by his courtesy name. He was from Changzhou, Jiangsu, was a salaried student in preparation for the imperial exam, and also conversant with Western learning. His initial occupation was teaching, and he quickly became a history instructor at the Teacher-Training Institute (*Shifan Jiangxisuo* 師範講習所). His *An Outline of Western History* (*Xishi gangmu* 西史綱目) enjoyed popularity. Later on, he moved to Shanghai and practiced medicine. In diagnosis and treatment, he used both Chinese and Western medicine, making him one of China's earliest doctors of integrated Chinese and Western medicine. After founding *Medical News*, Zhou Xueqiao then formed the Medical Research Association (*Yixue yanjiuhui* 醫學研究會), advocating the use of Chinese learning as the root and Western learning as the supplement to research the Chinese and Western medical arts. At the end of the thirty-first year of the *guangxu* reign period, he established the Chinese Medical

© KONINKLIJKE BRILL NV, LEIDEN, 2020 | DOI:10.1163/9789004420724_003

Association. For a while it received large numbers of members and attracted a good deal of publicity. *Medical News* also became the journal of the association. In the sixth month of the thirty-second year of the *guangxu* reign period, the famed gentleman Li Pingshu 李平書 along with the famous Shanghai physicians, Cai Xiaoxiang 蔡小香 and Gu Hongkui 顧鴻逵, initiated the establishment of the Shanghai Medical Association (*Shanghai yiwu zonghui* 上海醫務總會). Zhou Xueqiao was appointed one of the assistant managers to assist in the day-to-day affairs of this medical association. In organizing medical lectures and promoting Western medical knowledge, his contribution was tremendous. In the eighth month of the thirty-third year of the *guangxu* reign period, Zhou Xueqiao received an appointment and traveled north to Shanxi where he held the post of dean of studies at Shanxi Medical School (*Shanxi Yixue Guan* 山西醫學館) for about a year and a half. After he was resigned his post, he traveled to the capital where he remained for one year. Afterward he returned to Shanghai due to illness. In the second year of the *xuantong* reign period, he died of cancer.

Medical News is an example of a Chinese medical journal founded early in the modern period. All of the general methods of editing were established early on by Mr. Zhou. He repeatedly suffered setbacks and difficulties, but was able to bear it for eight years. It was truly not an easy task. When he first founded the journal, Xueqiao alone was personally responsible for all of the financial affairs and editing. In the summer of the thirty-second year of the *guangxu* reign period, when Mr. Zhou first received the invitation from Shanxi and went there to conclude the contract, he hoped to take responsibility for that province's medical instruction and intended to stop publishing *Medical News*. Because the influence of that journal extended over the entire country and had earned the esteem of the medical community, for a while famous physicians from all over wrote him numerous letters imploring him to stay. Moved by the feelings of so many people, Xueqiao remained in Shanghai and continued to issue the medical journal. In eighth month of the next year, after *Medical News* released its seventy-fourth issue, since he had repeatedly received earnest invitations from Shanxi, Xueqiao finally traveled north to take up the position and edited this journal from afar. However, he was cut off by mountain passes and postal service was inconvenient, so that the medical journal was frequently delayed. Xueqiao found the affairs of the Shanxi Medical School extremely onerous, and often he could not attend to one problem without neglecting another. Owing to these problems, at the end of the thirty-third year of the *guangxu* reign period, he took advantage of the opportunity of returning to Shanghai to celebrate Chinese New Year to ask Wang Wenqiao to take over running *Medical News.* Therefore, from the first day of the second month of the thirty-fourth year of the *guangxu* reign period, starting with the eightieth issue, Wang Wenqiao was the chief editor of *Medical News*, and the famous physician Cai Xiaoxiang was responsible for raising funds.

Wang Wenqiao (1873-?), whose given name was Zhen 槙, went by his courtesy name. He was from Shangyuan (modern Jiangning), Jiangsu, and was Cai Xiaoxiang's disciple. After taking over the management of *Medical News*, he obtained his teacher, Cai Xiaoxiang's, assistance in regard to finances. Cai allotted funds from the membership fees of the Chinese Medical Association. Wenqiao also invited Peng Banyu 彭伴漁, a member of the Chinese Medical Association, to manage the editing with him and Zheng Duanfu 鄭端甫, also a member, to assist in managing the affairs of the journal. In approximately the fifth month of the thirty-fourth year of the *guangxu* reign period, beginning with the eighty-seventh issue, he also invited Ding Fubao to join the editorial staff.

3. Shaoxing Medical Journal (Shaoxing yiyao xuebao 紹興醫藥學報)

In the sixth month of the thirty-fourth year of the *guangxu* reign period (1908), The *Shaoxing Medical Journal* was founded in Shaoxing by the Shaoxing Medical Association (*Shaoxing yiyao xuehui* 紹興醫藥學會). The Shaoxing Medical Research Society (*Shaoxing yiyaoxue yanjiushe* 紹興醫藥學研究社) were edited and were the primary distributors of the journal. The managers were the famous Shaoxing physicians, He Lianchen 何廉臣 and Qiu Jisheng 裘吉生. From its inception, this journal at times ceased publication for a variety of reasons. Among them, in the tenth month of the third year of the *xuantong* reign period (1911), due to political upheaval and "financial causes," the forty-fourth issue was released and then the journal shut down for almost four years. In July 1915, after the Shaoxing Medical Association changed names and became the Shaoxing branch of the Shenzhou Medical Association, the journal resumed publication (see, Cao Bingzhang 曹炳章, "Commemoration of the Anniversary of this Journal Resuming Publication [*Benbao jixu chuban zhounian jinianci* 本報繼續出版周年紀念辭]," volume 6, issue 1). After resuming publication, Qiu Jisheng became editor-in-chief. The journal was published through volume 13, number 1, and then ceased publication because Qiu Jisheng moved to Hangzhou. In total, it published 141 issues. From January 1910 onward, in addition to the journal, each week this periodical released the *Shaoxing Medical Journal Weekly Supplement* (*Shaoxing yiyaoxue bao xingqi zengkan* 紹興醫藥學報星期增刊). The *Shaoxing Medical Journal Weekly Supplement* altogether published 158 issues. Apart from being distributed in Shaoxing itself, there were distributers established in Hangzhou, Shanghai, Suzhou, and Nanjing.

He Lianchen (1861–1919), was named Bingyuan 炳元 and took the courtesy name Lianchen. He was born to a family of doctors in Shaoxing, Zhejiang. His paternal grandfather was the famous Shaoxing current cold damage expert, He Xiushan 何秀山. At first he applied himself to preparing for the imperial examination, but failed twice. He then shifted his focus to medicine and studied with the physicians Shen Liancha 沈蘭垞, Yan Jichun 嚴繼春, and Shen Yunchen 沈雲臣. He then followed the famous physician Fan Kaizhou 樊開周 in the clinic for three years. Afterwards, he traveled to Suzhou, Shanghai, and Shaoxing, seeking the principles of medicine from the famous physicians Ma Peizhi 馬培之 and Zhao Qingchu 趙晴初. Together with Zhou Xueqiao and Ding Fubao, he began the formation of the Chinese Medical Association (*Zhongguo*

© KONINKLIJKE BRILL NV, LEIDEN, 2020 | DOI:10.1163/9789004420724_004

yixuehui 中國醫學會). Before the thirty-third year of the *guangxu* reign period, he traveled to Japan and came into contact with Western medicine. He purchased a wide range of Western medical books and advocated for the harmonious blending of Chinese and Western medicine. Following the thirty-fourth year of the *guangxu* reign period. Following the thirty-fourth year of the *guangxu* reign period, he practiced medicine privately in Shaoxing. Mr. He inwardly drew on the ancient and the modern and outwardly brought together the Chinese and the Western. His learning was deep and broad. He promoted the practical and had no use for the merely showy. He opposed empty talk that was mired in the ancient. He decided to form a medical association because he was distressed by the decline of the medical community and the difficulty of practicing medicine. He advocated researching both Eastern and Western medicine and edited a medical journal in order to exchange knowledge and experience and also to provide guidance for the nation's people.

Qiu Jisheng (1873–1947) was originally named Qingyuan 慶元. His original courtesy name was Jisheng 激聲. He later changed it to Jisheng. He was from Shaoxing, Zhejiang. In his youth, he joined the anti-Qing Restoration League (*Guangfu hui* 光復會) and United League (*Tongmeng hui* 同盟會). He used medical practice as a cover for engaging in revolutionary activities. Later on, having traveled to Shenyang and contacted people in the Revolutionary Party, he became acquainted with Japanese medical personages and extensively collected Han medicine (*Hanyi* 漢醫) texts from at home and abroad. Following the 1911 Revolution, he returned to Shaoxing, roused the medical association from slumber, reinvigorated the medical journal, and opened a hospital. In 1921, he moved to Hangzhou where he established the Triple-Three Medical Society (*San-san yishe* 三三醫社), published medical books, and founded the *Triple-Three Medical Journal* (*San-san yibao* 三三醫報). While actively in exploring the principles of medicine and at the same time emphasizing clinical practice, Mr. Qiu even more energetically pushed forward the development of medical theory and medical treatment. By establishing a hospital, founding a medical journal, and editing and publishing Chinese and foreign medical books, he contributed to the broad spread of medical knowledge and hastened the advance of socialist medicine.

4. The International Medical Journal (Zhongxi yixue bao 中西醫學報)

On the fifteenth day of the fourth month of the second year of the *xuantong* reign period (May 23rd, 1910), *The International Medical Journal*[1] was founded in Shanghai. This journal was a monthly periodical. Ding Fubao was the editor-in-chief. It was edited and published by the Shanghai Chinese-Western Medical Research Association (*Shanghai Zhong-Xi yixue yanjiuhui* 上海中西醫學研究會). The principle location for distribution was established at 81 Changshou Settlement, Xinma Road, Shanghai. The journal was printed in a 32mo printing format up to July, 1918. Its purpose was to "introduce medical learning, propagate the true principles of hygiene, and to cultivate consummate human virtue and sound judgment" ("Notice to Readers [*Jinggao duzhe* 敬告讀者]," volume 9, number 1). In July 1918, "Because Mr. Ding Fubao is compiling *Glosses of Words in the Explanation of Graphs (Shuowen gulin* 說文詁林), in over one thousand sections, he has no time for other projects. Therefore, the medical journal must announce a temporary halt in publication. In January 1927, it resumed publication under the management of Ding Fubao's son, Ding Huikang 丁惠康. It still continued to use the name *International Medical Journal* without change, but the printing format was changed to 16mo ("The Evolution of this Journal," in *Flourishing Virtue Medical Journal* [*Dehua yixue zazhi* 德華醫學雜誌], number 1). In 1928, this journal name was changed to *Flourishing Virtue Medical Journal* by Ding Mingquan 丁名全, who graduated from a German university.[2] Ding Yangkang 丁錫康, who had graduated from Shanghai's St. John's University medical course, assisted with the editing. The journal was located at 121 Baige Road, Shanghai and was distributed principally by Medicine Press (*Yixue shuju* 醫學書局). The purpose of the journal was to, "adopt the approach of making learning widely available in order to disseminate the new medicine and accelerate the realization of public health" ("Editor's Note, [*Bianzhe yan* 編者言]" *Flourishing Virtue Medical Journal*, volume 1, number 1). The *Flourishing Virtue Medical Journal* published altogether one volume and twelve issues. In June, 1929, it again changed names, restoring the original title,

---

1 A literal translation of the journal's title would be "*Chinese-Western Medical Journal*" but the journal itself used the English title "*The International Medical Journal*."

2 *Translator's Note*: 衛慈堡大學, possibly the University of Würzburg, but the identification is uncertain. The name of the journal may also be a play on words, as it could also be read as the "German-Chinese Medical Journal."

© KONINKLIJKE BRILL NV, LEIDEN, 2020 | DOI:10.1163/9789004420724_005

International Medical Journal. It also continued the numbering of the original series, starting at volume 10, number 1. After publishing the twelfth volume, it ceased publication. From its founding to June, 1930, *International Medical Journal* published a total of 132 issues.

Ding Fubao (1874–1952) used the courtesy name Zhonggu 仲祜 as well as the courtesy name Meixuan 梅軒. He used the sobriquet Chouyinjushi 疇隱居士. He was from Wuxi, Jiangsu. He studied at Jiangyin Nanjing Academy (*Jiangyin Nanjing shuyuan* 江陰南菁書院). Later, he entered in Suzhou's Dongwu University (*Dongwu daxue* 東吳大學). In the twenty-seventh year of the *guangxu* reign period of the Qing dynasty (1901), he further enrolled in Shanghai's Dongwen School (*Dongwen xuetang* 東文學堂) to study Japanese and medicine. At the age of twenty-six, having suffered from prolonged illness, he devoted himself to medicine, taking Zhao Yuanyi as his teacher 趙元益. Zhao Yuanyi was a famous physician of the time. He had insights into physiology, anatomy, pharmacy, and health preservation from both Chinese and Western perspective and had translated and written introductions to modern Western medical texts. He may well be said to have deeply penetrated Chinese and Western medicine. This caused Ding Fubao to develop a deep understanding of both Chinese and Western medicine. In the twenty-ninth year of the *guangxu* reign period, he accepted Zhang Zhidong's 張之洞 offer of a position and moved to the capital to take charge of teaching mathematics and physiology at the Translation Institute of the Imperial University (*Daxuetang yixueguan* 大學堂譯學館). In the thirtieth year of the *guangxu* reign period, when the Chinese Medical Association (*Zhongguo yixue hui* 中國醫學會) was established, he became its vice-president. In the pages of that association's journal, *Medical News* (*Yixue bao* 醫學報), he frequently wrote articles introducing Western knowledge of anatomy and physiology. In the first year of the *xuantong* reign period in the medical exams of the Imperial Inspectorate held in Nanjing, he obtained the "Outstanding Internal Medicine Physician" certificate, earning the respect of Duan Fang 端方 and Sheng Xuanhuai 盛宣懷. He was appointed to proceed to Japan to research medicine. After returning to China in the second year of the *xuantong* reign period, he established the Chinese-Western Medicine Research Association (*Zhong-Xi yixue yanjiuhui* 中西醫學研究會), gathering together his colleagues in the Chinese-Western medical world, advocating for medical research, and publishing the association's research in *International Medical Journal.* In diagnosing illnesses, Ding Fubao chose to use modern Western medical methods of diagnosis—using physical and chemical examinations as well as x-rays and microscopy—in order to verify the diagnosis and be certain the medicine fit the syndrome. He established a medical publishing house, a hospital, and a sanatorium.

He edited, translated, and published Japanese-language Western medical books. He introduced the our country's medical profession to Western medical knowledge and accelerated the cultural interchange between China and Japan (Yi Guangqian 伊廣謙, "A Brief Description of Ding Fubao's Life and Writings [*Ding Fubao shengping ji qi zhuzuo shulue* 丁福保生平及其著作述略]," *Understanding Medical Writings in Classical Chinese* [*Yiguwen zhishi* 醫古文知識], 2003, number 1). In 1939, he accepted an invitation to become editor-in-chief of *New Approaches to National Medicinals* 國藥新聲.

Ding Huikang (1904–1979) was heavily influenced by his father from his childhood onward. After graduating from high school, he devoted himself to medicine. In 1911, he graduated from Shanghai's Tongji Medical University (*Tongji yike daxue* 同濟醫科大學) and immediately took over the resumed publication of the *International Medical Journal*. In Shanghai, he established a sanatorium for lung diseases and the Hongqiao Sanatorium. Throughout his life he admired and collected cultural relics. After the founding of the People's Republic of China, he was appointed a consultant to the Shanghai city cultural relics management committee and a member of the Shanghai Cultural History Research Institute.

5. Shenzhou Medical Journal (Shenzhou yiyaoxue bao 神州醫藥學報)

In May of 1911 (the second year of the Republican Period), the *Shenzhou*[1] *Medical Journal* was founded in Shanghai by the Shenzhou Medical Association (*Shenzhou yiyao zonghui* 神州醫藥總會) with Yu Botao 余伯陶 as editor. At the start of publication, it was set as a monthly periodical. It was published on the fifteenth or sixteenth day of the month, according to the lunar calendar, in a 32mo printing format. In January of 1915, after publishing the thirtieth issue, it ceased publication. In October 1923, it resumed publication, but its publication schedule was not fixed. In April 1925, it again ceased publication, having published six issues. After it resumed publication, the specific arrangements were all taken care of by Bao Shisheng 包識生. Mr. Bao accepted a position at the Suzhou Epidemiology Institute (*Suzhou shiyi yuan* 蘇州時疫院); therefore, from volume two, issue 4 onward, he did not manage the details of editing and publication, but he still articles in the journal. In 1921, the Shenzhou Medical Association changed its name to the Shenzhou National Medicine Association (*Shenzhou guoyi xuehui* 神州國醫學會) and in 1932 began publication of the *Shenzhou Journal of National Medicine* (*Shenzhou guoyi xuebao* 神州國醫學報).

The numbering of volumes and issues for this journal contains inconsistencies. The first twenty-five issues are numbered year 1, issues 1–7, year 2, issues 1–12, and year 3, issues 1–6. The remaining issues are numbered issues 26–30. After resuming publication the issues were numbered volume 2, issues 1–6. In the first year, each issue was forty-eight to seventy pages in length. From the second year onward, the quantity of content expanded, and the number of pages increased, reaching eighty to 126 pages.

Regarding the causes of the cessation and resumption of publication, "An Announcement by Bao Shisheng," in volume 2, issue 1, "owing to several years of financial difficulties, I didn't have the strength to keep going. I had no choice but to proceed gradually, halt publication, and wait for there to be others who wished to restore the prestige of the learning of the Yellow Emperor and the Divine Husbandman (*Huang-Nong zhi xue* 黃農之學). To my surprise, the wait stretched to eight years. When one sat down to discuss it, it was certainly not the case that there was no one interested, but when one arose to do it, there was actually no one to be seen." Mr. Bao worried that Chinese medicine was

---

1 *Translator's Note*: Literally, "the Divine Land," a poetic way of referring to China.

in an urgent state where time was of the essence. Therefore, he once again assembled the medical world's physicians of great talent and vast learning to "rouse the troops after a defeat." From the time of its founding the distribution site for this journal changed incessantly. The earliest location was in Ankang Settlement, Paoma Creek, Shanghai. Later on it moved to Bao'an Settlement, Xiaohua Garden, Sanma Road, then to Beitingji Settlement, Lao Lajiqiao creek, and then to Qipu Intersection, North Zhejiang Road. The difficulty of publication is revealed by the rather large number of changes.

The editor-in-chief, Yu Botao (1872–1945) used the courtesy name Dexun. He was from Jiading, Jiangsu. As a child he immersed himself in the classics, the histories, and the various schools of thought from the pre-Qin period. As a youth he studied medicine with Chen Ziran 陳子然 from Suzhou. His learning was deep and broad. He was particularly adept at cold damage and seasonal epidemics. His published writings include *Revealing the Secrets of Plague* (*Shuyi juewei* 鼠疫抉微), *Collected Discussions on Epidemic Patterns* (*Yizheng jishuo* 疫證集說), *The Ancient Meaning of Cold Damage* (*Shanghan guyi* 傷寒古義). He was also skilled at writing poetry, authoring the *Huaiyuan Hall Collection* (*Huaiyuan tang ji* 懷遠堂集). At various points he was the vice-president of the Shanghai United Medical Association (*Shanghai yiyao lianhe hui* 上海醫藥聯合會) and a trustee of the Shanghai Medical Services Association (*Shanghai yiwu zonghui* 上海醫務總會). Because the ministry of education emphasized Western medical knowledge, he invited like-minded individuals from every province to form the Shenzhou Medical Association and was elected its president. He traveled north to look into the matter, protect the national essence, and preserve the learning of the *Numinous Pivot* (*Lingshu* 靈樞) and *Basic Questions* (*Suwen* 素問). He succeeded in obtaining government approval and enjoyed prestige within the medical profession (*Biographical Sketches* [*Zhuanlue* 傳略], volume 2, number 4).

Bao Shisheng, (ca. 1874–1934) was named Yixu 一虛 and used the courtesy name Dedai 德逮. He was from Shanghang, Fujian. He was born in a family of hereditary Chinese medical doctors. His father, Bao Taochu, was skilled in the study of cold damage. When treating illnesses he did not use modern medicinal formulae, but instead used modifications of classical formulae. Shisheng was his oldest son. From childhood he inherited the family learning and revered classical medicinal formulae. He diligently studied the [*Treatise on*] *Cold Damage and Miscellaneous Diseases* (*Shanghan zabing* 傷寒雜病) for ten years and grasped the subtleties of Changsha [Zhang Zhongjing].[2] At the age

---

2   Zhang Ji 張機 (ca. 150–219), better known by his courtesy name Zhongjing 仲景, wrote the extremely influential medical text *Treatise on Cold Damage and Miscellaneous Diseases*

of twenty he began to receive patients on his own and earned an excellent reputation. In 1911 he moved to Shanghai. Afterwards, he founded the *Shenzhou Medical Journal* with Yu Botao. Mr. Bao alone contributed more than sixty articles to this journal. In 1918, the Shenzhou Specialized Medical Training School (*Shenzhou yiyao zhuanke xuexiao* 神州醫藥專科學校) was founded, and Mr. Bao became the Dean of Studies. However, because it was strapped for funds, this school closed shortly thereafter. In 1928, he became an instructor at the Shanghai Chinese Medicine Institute (*Shanghai Zhongguo yixue yuan* 上海中國醫學院) where he participated in the production of teaching materials and trained the next generation of Chinese medical talent. His writings were mostly about Zhongjing theory. He authored *The Treatise on Cold Damage by Chapters and Sections* (*Shanghan lun zhangjie* 傷寒論章節) and *Teaching Materials on the Treatise on Cold Damage* (*Shanghan lun jiangyi* 傷寒論講義). All of his writings were gathered together in three collections, titled *Mr. Bao's Collected Medical Works* (*Baoshi yizong* 包氏醫宗).

Yu Botao founded the Shenzhou Medical Association because, in the first year of the Republican period, "the ministry of education left out the proposal about Chinese medicine." After its founding, he visited the capital two times to look into the matter and put it on record through the approval of the state council's ministries of internal affairs and education (Xu Xiangchen 徐相宸, *Lectures in the Vernacular* 白話演講, volume 1, issue 1). *Shenzhou Medical Journal* was the Shenzhou Medical Association's journal. It came into being along with the birth of this association. The two of them supplemented and completed one another and were inextricably linked. "Concise Regulations for the Formation of the Shenzhou Medical Association (*Chouban Shenzhou yiyao zonghui jianzhang* 籌辦神州醫藥總會簡章)," in the journal's inaugural issue, established the name, Shenzhou Medical Association, and set its general aim as "connecting the medical circles of each province, advancing the accomplishments of research, and protecting the intrinsic national essence in order to develop our noble and exquisite medical heritage passed down from the Yellow Emperor and Qibo and strive for the public's health." It also spelled out in detail the association's office, its members, its powers, and its fees. The "Concise Regulations" clearly stipulated, "the office of president is temporarily left vacant until it can be filled by a worthy candidate. When the winds moving

---

(*Shanghan zabing lun* 傷寒雜病論) ca. 206. It now only exists as two separate texts: the *Treatise on Cold Damage* (*Shanghan lun* 傷寒論) and *Essentials of the Golden Coffer* (*Jingui yaolue* 金匱要略). They remain an essential study for all doctors of Chinese herbal medicine to this day, and were at the center of the debates about modernization of Chinese medicine in the early 20th century.

over the seas assemble the talented individuals, we will then open a formal association and vote to elect a president in clear solemnity." In the early stages of the founding of the association, Yu Botao, Ding Ganren 丁甘仁, and Qian Xiangyuan 錢庠元 took charge of directing the association and managing its finances. Wang Wenqiao 王問樵 acted as general secretary. There was also a secretary in charge of documents, a discussant, a secretary cum correspondent, a secretary for meeting minutes, an accountant cum business manager, and an investigator. The association had fifty-six honorary members such as Cen Chunxuan 岑春煊, Cai Jimin 蔡濟民, Zhang Mingqi 張鳴岐, and Zhu Xiaonan 朱曉南. The 668 regular members included Lu Jinsheng 陸晉笙, Xu Xiangchen, Bao Shisheng, and Xu Xiaopu 徐小圃 and were located both north and south of the Yangtze and even overseas. Its influence was profound and far-reaching.

The "Forward to the Journal" written by Yu Botao states that in the spring of the *gui-chou* year like-minded individuals formed the Shenzhou Medical Association. That summer, they published their official journal (*Shenzhou Medical Journal*): "to take responsibility for leading all of the entire nation's medical profession." The article argues that in the twentieth century, there was not one among the great powers that did not compete fiercely. If China's medical science relaxes even a bit, there was a danger of regression. If they wanted to survive, research and reform were necessary. This journal, "cannot bear to miss this opportunity" and "wishes to maintain connections with all of the broadly talented individuals throughout the country." It shouldered the task of preserving the national essence and "focuses on medical research" "not on the conflicts and dissension of the various schools of thought." "Someday, the great physicians of our country's medicine will be able, on the vast stage of the world, to shine forth with a great light. I cannot help but pray sincerely for that day" ("Forward to the Journal," year 1, issue 1).

6. Medical Magazine (Yixue zazhi 醫學雜誌)

In June 1921 (the tenth year of the Republican period), *Medical Magazine* was founded in Taiyuan, Shanxi. It was established by the Taiyuan-Shanxi Chinese Medical Improvement Research Association (*Shanxi Taiyuan zhongyi gaijin yanjiuhui* 山西太原中醫改進研究會). It was published bimonthly in a 32mo printing format. On November 8th, 1937, Japanese soldiers occupied Taiyuan, and the magazine was forced to cease publication. Over the course of sixteen years, it published ninety-six issues. It was one of the earliest, broadest in scope of publishing, and longest-running medical journals in the country.

In April 1919, seeing that it would not be easy at the time to widely disseminate Western medicine, the military cum civil governor of the Shanxi, Yan Yangshan 閻錫山, initiated the establishment of the Shanxi Chinese Medicine Improvement Research Association (hereafter, the Improvement Association). Initially they provisionally managed the association's affairs from the meeting room in the western building of the military governor's mansion. One year later, they moved to Xinmin Street. In order to demonstrate the importance he placed on this association, Yan Yangshan himself took the position of president. The then brigade commander Zhao Daiwen 趙戴文 took the post of honorary director-general. The head of governmental affairs, Yang Zhaotai 楊兆泰 became the director-general. The seventeen directors included Zhang Siqing 張思卿, Yin Qingyuan 陰慶元, Chen Guanguang 陳觀光, Li Yuanchang 李垣昌, and Ding Lanquan 丁蘭泉. The research association also specified that it would not accept limitations as to the number of people who could join. They invited honorary directors from the entire medical community of China. Nearly one hundred famous physicians from all across the country—including each of the fourteen provincial-level cities—were invited to become honorary directors, including Ding Fubao 丁福報, Xu Shangzhi 徐尚志, Xue Baochen 薛寶宸, Xiao Yanping 蕭延平, and Ma Deji 馬德基. This caused the Chinese medical profession in Shanxi to experience a rather brilliant period of development. The research association extensively recruited members both inside and outside of the province. Through its membership system, the research association brought together large numbers of talented physicians from across the country. In 1937, on the eve of its disintegration, the research association had approximately one thousand members. It had a significant impact on the Chinese medical community of that period.

Recognizing that at that time the country revered Western medicine and looked down on Chinese medicine, this association took "improving Chinese medicine and pharmacology and enabling it to become a high-level system of learning as its purpose" (Constitution of the Chinese Medicine Improvement Research Association, section 1). In its inaugural issue, this journal published a public address by Yan Yangshan. He put forward an opposing view in regard to the contemporary situation of Chinese and Western medicine and clearly explained original intention and purpose behind the establishment of the Improvement Association. To summarize, he stated that he hoped the Improvement Association could make a contribution in three areas that would supplement the medical capacity so desperately needed by the common people: first, supporting our nation's production of Chinese medicinals; second, helping to eliminate the current state of affairs in which the common people lack both physicians and medicinals; and third, countering the current exorbitant price of Western drugs.

This journal emphasized explorations and expositions of the essence of medicine from the point of view of Chinese and Western medicine. It also put forward as its purpose for publication: "Developing the true principles of Chinese medicine, consulting and verifying them by Western medical science, get to the heart of the matter by seeking the source, and achieve mastery by comprehensive study." Due to having suffered the impact and influence of Western culture, the flowing together of Chinese and Western thought flourished throughout the country. In this context, this journal took improving and advancing the development of Chinese medicine as its goal. Emphasizing excavating the theory and traditional treatment methods of Chinese medicine, it gradually gave expression to the special character of an all-inclusive coming together of the Chinese and Western. The magazine published many of the contemporary medical community's advanced treatises and proved very influential.

7. *Shanghai's* Chinese Medicine Magazine (Zhongyi zazhi 中醫雜誌) (*including Shanghai's* National Medicine Magazine [Guoyi zazhi 國醫雜誌])

On January 12th, 1922, (the eleventh year of the Republican period), *Chinese Medicine Magazine* was founded in Shanghai by Wang Yiren 王一仁, Dai Dafu 戴大夫, and Qin Bowei 秦伯未. Wang Yiren was the editor-in-chief. It was the journal of the Shanghai Chinese Medical Association (*Shanghai zhongyi xuehui* 上海中醫學會). It was published quarterly and sold throughout the country and even as far overseas as Singapore, Japan, and America. It was one of the most influential Chinese medical periodicals of the Republican period. In the summer of 1918, Wang Yiren left Shanghai for Zhejiang and the editorship was taken over by Cheng Menxue 程門雪 and Yu Hongsun 余鴻孫. Chen Tiandun 陳天鈍 assisted with the editorial work.

In September of 1930 the thirtieth issue was published. On October 27th, the Committee for Training the People of the Nationalist government's party headquarters for the special city of Shanghai ordered the association to cease all activities, claiming that "the organization's name is fantastic and its organization unsuitable." This journal, therefore, ceased publication. In July of the next year, after the Shanghai Chinese Medical Association had persuaded the authorities to register it, it underwent a reorganization. After the reorganization, its name was changed to Shanghai National Medicine Trade Association (*Shanghai shi guoyi gonghui* 上海市國醫公會). Zhou Shaonan 周召南 became director of the association's editorial department and Yu Shunchen 虞舜臣 became editor of the magazine. In November, the magazine resumed publication under the name *Chinese Medicine Magazine*. The issue numbers continued the previous series, starting with issue 31. At the end of the month this same issue was reprinted under the changed name *National Medicine Magazine*, issue 1.

When *Chinese Medicine Magazine*, the plan envisaged was to "temporarily use a quarterly publication as a model then gradually advance to a monthly and then weekly publication" ("Notes," *Chinese Medicine Magazine*, issue 1), but as of September 1930, there had actually been no "advance" toward a monthly publication. After its name was changed to *National Medicine Magazine*, [the editors] again declared that "we should make this quarterly publication into a monthly publication, so that the association's members will profit greatly" (Yu Shunchen, "This Journal Going Forward," *National Medicine Magazine*, issue 1), but they were also ultimately unable to realize their wishes. The difficulties

© KONINKLIJKE BRILL NV, LEIDEN, 2020 | DOI:10.1163/9789004420724_008

were all the result of insufficient funding. Because the first issue of *National Medicine Magazine* was a reprint of issue 31 of *Chinese Medicine Magazine*, it was published on November 31st [*sic*], 1931, at the same time as issue 2. Issues 3 and 4 were published separately in June and December of 1932. Starting with the publication of issue 5—on March 31, 1933—the journal returned more or less to the publishing schedule of the prior *Chinese Medicine Magazine*, publishing according to the pattern of spring, summer, autumn, and winter.

After the sudden outbreak of the War of Resistance against Japan, Shanghai fell into enemy hands, and the Shanghai National Medicine Trade Association was forced to halt of its activities. The magazine also ceased publication at that time. In August 1946, the National Medicine Trade Association resumed its activities which continued until its formal dissolution in 1951. Because it underwent many years of tribulations and setbacks, it is difficult to calculate accurately the amount of time the *National Medicine Magazine* was out of print and the number of issues it published. The latest issue the author has seen was issue 31.

8. Triple-Three Medical Journal (San-san yibao 三三醫報)

In July 1923 (the twelfth year of the Republican period), *Triple-Three Medical Journal* was founded in Hangzhou. This journal was released every ten days in a "large overseas-style quarto format." Publication was suspended every summer for the month of July, so every year thirty-three issues were released. Altogether it published four volumes and 132 issues. Qiu Jisheng 裘吉生 was both the president of the Triple-Three Medical Journal Society and the journal's editor. Qiu Jisheng explained his reason for choosing the name *Triple-Three Medical Journal*: "Doctors need to read the books of the three generations and seek for three year-old artemisia, only then will they be able to break their arm three times.[1] Therefore, I have chosen this name" ("*Triple-Three Medical Journal's Purpose* [*San-san yibao dazhi* 三三醫報大旨]," volume 1, issue 1).

Qiu Jisheng (1873–1947) was originally named Qingyuan 慶元 and used the courtesy-name Jisheng. He was from Shaoxing, Zhejiang. In his youth he joined the anti-Qing Restoration Party (*Guangfu hui* 光復會). Later, having left Shaoxing and moved to Shanghai, he joined the Revolutionary Alliance, using his practice of medicine as a cover for his continued revolutionary activities. When he traveled to Shenyang to make contact with the members of Revolutionary Party, he had the opportunity to get to know people from the Japanese medical community and became devoted to collecting rare and valuable medical texts. He sought out and purchased Chinese medical texts (*Hanyi shuji* 漢醫書籍)[2] from abroad, Japanese printings of Chinese medical texts, and hand-written manuscripts left behind by worthy authors of the past. He obtained numerous precious old editions and exquisitely written manuscripts. After the triumph of the 1911 Revolution, he returned to his native place and practiced medicine in Suzhou. Mr. Qiu habitually placed great emphasis on medical ethics and enjoyed an excellent reputation in the medical

---

1   The "books of the three generations" refer to ancient medical books on acupuncture, medicinal therapy, and pulse diagnosis. "three year-old artemisia" is a reference to chapter 7 of the classic *Mencius*, Mencius states, "… in treating a seven year-old illness, you seek for three year-old artemisia." Artemisia is the plant that is used to produce moxa, a wooly substance burned to heat points on the body as a medical treatment. Older artemisia plants are said to make stronger medicine. "Breaking their arm three times" is a traditional metaphor for gaining valuable experience through difficult experiences.

2   Literally "Han medicine texts." Here, this refers to texts on Chinese medicine produced outside of China.

community. In 1915, Mr. Qiu formed the Shaoxing branch of the Shenzhou Medical Association (*Shenzhou yixue hui Shaoxing fenhui* 神州醫學會紹興分會) and assumed its presidency. In little time, he had resumed publication of the *Shaoxing Medical Journal* (*Shaoxing yixue bao* 紹興醫學報) (this journal had ceased publication in 1911) and become its editor-in-chief. Through the combined efforts of Qiu Jisheng and the like-minded He Lianchen 何廉臣 and Cao Bingzhang 曹炳章, that journal's scholarly activity was extraordinarily vigorous. The nations famous physicians, such as Zhang Yangdun 張錫頓 and Zhang Shanlei 張山雷, all published articles in this journal, making it one of the Chinese medical community's important scholarly arenas. In 1921, Qiu Jisheng moved to Hangzhou, established the Triple-Three Medical Society (*San-san yishe* 三三醫社) and published medical books. He continued to produce periodicals, founding the *Triple-Three Medical Journal*. He also opened the Triple-Three Hospital, which had physicians practicing both Chinese and Western medicine. Patients who were suitable for Western medical treatment, they used Western methods; those suitable for Chinese medicine took Chinese medicinals. For patients with severe and dangerous illnesses, the Chinese and Western medical physicians consulted together. In 1929, Mr. Qiu was the representative for Zhejiang at the Shanghai Assembly. He protested the draft resolution: "Abolish Chinese Medicine," and personally joined the resistance movement going to Nanjing to present a petition to the national government. He vigorously rushed about in order to protect Chinese medicine.

9. Shaoxing Medical Monthly (Shaoxing yiyao yuebao 紹興醫藥月報)

In January 1924 (the thirteenth year of the Republican period), *Shaoxing Medical Monthly* was founded in Shaoxing by He Lianchen 何廉臣 and Cao Bingzhang 曹炳章—the then president of the Shaoxing branch of the Shenzhou Medical Association (*Shenzhou yixuehui Shaoxing fenhui* 神州醫學會紹興分會) and the head of the supervisory committee of the Shaoxing Chinese-Western Medical Association (*Shaoxing Zhong-Xi yi xiehui* 紹興中西醫協會). respectively—who, together with She Tongjia 社同甲, invited like-minded people to pool their capital and found it. She Tongjia was the editor-in-chief. He Lianchen was the assistant editor. The more than twenty editors included Zhou Yuege 周越鉻, Yang Zhi'an 楊質安, Hu Baoshu 胡寶書, and Fu Boyang 傅伯揚. The journal sought the endorsement of more than thirty famous physicians as honorary members, including Zhang Yangchun 張錫純, Zhang Taiyan 張太炎, Zhou Xiaonong 周小農, Yun Tieqiao 惲鐵樵, and Shi Mianren 時逸人.

In November 1926, after publishing its thirty-fifth issue, this journal ceased publication for seven months. The following year in July, it resumed publication with its thirty-sixth issue (volume 3, issue 12). After that, due to He Lianchen's age and infirmity, it again ceased publication, this time for three months. In September of the same year, at the suggestion of the original editor-in-chief, She Tongjia, the journal returned to auspices of the Shaoxing Chinese-Western Medicine Association and resumed publication. He Youlian 何幼廉, Chen Yichen 陳儀臣, Cao Bingzhang, and Qiu Shidong 裘士東 became the editors and continuously posted changing announcements on the first page of the journal. In November, they published the thirty-seventh issue (volume 4, number 1) and then published twelve issues without interruption. They stopped publication in October of the following year, having reached the forty-ninth issue.

He Lianchen (1861–1929) was named Bingyuan 炳元 and used the sobriquet Yinyan 印岩, meaning "confirming Ye Xiangyan's 葉香岩 theories."[1] In his later years he called himself "the decrepit old man from eastern Zhejiang (*Yuezhong laoxiu* 越中老朽)." He was from Shaoxing, Zhejiang, and was a famous Chinese medical physician at the end of the Qing and the beginning of the Republican

---

1 Ye Xiangyan, named Ye Gui 葉桂, and best known by his courtesy name Tianshi 天士 was a tremendously influential 18th century doctor.

period. He practiced medicine for over fifty years. He compiled *Categorized Proven Cases of Famous Physicians from the Entire Country (Quanguo mingyi yan'an leibian* 全國名醫驗案類編), in order to standardize case histories for seasonal illnesses. He also wrote *A Compendium of Patterns and Treatment for Internal Medicine (Neike zhengzhi quanshu* 內科證治全書). He Lianchen was historically located in precisely the period of time during which China transitioned from a feudal society to a modern society. Following the invasion of the Western Great Powers, there was a massive influx of Western cultural ideas that produced a tremendous impression on Chinese society. The import of Western medicine also made a huge impact on Chinese medicine. In order to save and develop Chinese medicine, He Lianchen exerted himself in forming Chinese medical organizations and managing Chinese medical periodicals. He sought to strengthen the exchange of knowledge in order to protect and develop Chinese medicine so that it could make its important contribution. He Lianchen revered Chinese medicine, advocated for the unification of Chinese and Western medicine, and when appropriate absorbed the new knowledge of Western medicine in order to vigorously develop Chinese medicine. In August 1909, when the "Shaoxing Medical Research Society" formed (the following year its name was changed to "Shaoxing Medical Association"), became and remained its president. With his support, the *Shaoxing Medical Journal (Shaoxing yiyao xuebao* 紹興醫藥學報) and the *Shaoxing Medical Monthly* were successively founded and published.

In July 1909, *Shaoxing Medical Journal* was founded in Shaoxing. In January 1923, that journal published volume 13, number 1 (issue 143). Afterward—since the then editor-in-chief, Qiu Jisheng, moved to Hangzhou—it ceased publication. When *Shaoxing Medical Monthly* was founded, it remained essentially oriented to the same purpose as *Shaoxing Medical Journal*, taking "expounding ancient learning, introducing of new knowledge, and vigorously striving for medical progress, all for the sake of aiding our ill compatriots" as purpose for publication ("Constitution of the Shaoxing Medical Monthly Society [*Shaoxing yiyao yuebao she jianzhang* 紹興醫藥月報社簡章]," volume 1, issue 1), as well as proposing the scientization of medicine, putting forward the need to refashion Chinese medicine, and advocating for searching for connections with Western medicine. In the inaugural issue of *Shaoxing Medical Monthly*, He Lianchen published this journal's manifesto: "Therefore, with all humbleness and sincerity, I ask my compatriots far and wide to first test our country's historical medical theory to see what is worthy and what is unworthy, what must be discarded and what can be followed, so that each of you may develop individual clinical realizations about the reality of clinical practice. Following the example of science, categorize, compile, and write about it. Discus it with the skilled doctors of the entire country. Go in search of criticism. Urge our country's medicine forward in expectation of the time when it will, in company with all the other branches of science, arrive at a noble and enlightened realm" ("A Declaration of this Journal's Purpose [*Benbao zongzhi zhi xuanyan* 本報宗旨之宣言]," volume 1, number 1).

For a period of time, as the esteem of Western studies advanced eastward, Western medicine was transmitted to our country, and foreigners established hospitals in China, Chinese medicine took a beating. Added to this, a culture of fondness for the new and disgust with the old was on the rise in the society of the time. Influenced by this culture, some people lashed out at Chinese medicine. They saw Chinese medicine as an old and outworn field of knowledge. "Since Western medicine—with its strength to topple mountains and overturn seas—made incursions into our country, the disciples of uplifting the Western and repressing the Chinese always seize upon one or two errors in Chinese medical texts and then generalize to the totality of Chinese medicine, saying it is not worth even a single glance" ("Appendix to the Notice Sent to the Ministry of Education [*Fulu shang jiaoyubu gongwen* 附錄上教育部公文]," volume 2, number 10). In order to save and develop Chinese medicine, He Lianchen stridently opened up a new avenue of development for Chinese medicine. He emphasized mastering both the ancient and the modern, absorbing new knowledge, and setting up medical education. He said, "If our method of using indications and other theories can be explained by the new and advanced science, then Chinese medicine's newness and uniqueness will be irrefutable. How can one speak of 'old and outworn?' How can one use the single phrase 'old and outworn' to write off at one stroke the achievements of the experience of the famous physicians of from antiquity to modern times?" ("A Declaration of this Journal's Purpose [*Benbao zongzhi zhi xuanyan* 本報宗旨之宣言]," volume 1, number 1).

10. Shenyang Medical Magazine (Shenyang yixue zazhi 瀋陽醫學雜誌)

In the autumn of 1924 (the thirteenth year of the Republican Period), *Shenyang Medical Magazine* was founded in Shenyang by Ma Yinglin 馬英麟 and Shen Wenkui 沈文魁. It was published by the Shenyang Medical Society (*Shenyang yixue she* 瀋陽醫學社). Zhang Yangchun 張錫純 and Liu Jingsu 劉景素 were the editors-in-chief. Zhang Zhiliang 張志良 wrote the journal title and the title of the various columns in his calligraphy. Immediately upon publishing the fourth issue, the journal ceased publication due to the Zhi-Feng War (*Zhi-Feng zhanzheng* 直奉戰爭)[1] and Zhang Yangchun returning to his native village. Later on, with the support of the newly-founded Fengtian Physician's Trade Association (*Fengtian yishi gonghui* 奉天醫士公會) (Zhang Zhiliang was president), the resumed publication of the fifth issue. It was now published by the Fengtian Physicians Trade Association. Liu Jingsu became the research department chief. Shen Wenkui and Ma Yinglin became the editors-in-chief. After publishing the seventh issue in April 1925, the journal's name was changed to *Fengtian Physician's Magazine* (*Fengtian yishi zazhi* 奉天醫士雜誌) in order to make it match the name "Fengtian Physician's Trade Association." This journal was oriented toward distribution throughout the entire country, but owing to difficulties in transportation, its distribution was concentrated in Shenyang. Moreover, its target audience was primarily the members of the Fengtian Physician's Trade Association. For five years, the journal continued to be published on the tenth of each month, publishing ten issues every year (no issues were published during the first and last lunar month of each year). Afterwards, due to increasing turmoil and violence as well as economic difficulties, it was forced to cease publication in March 1928, after publishing the twenty-sixth issue.

Zhang Yangchun (1860–1933) used the courtesy name Shoufu 壽甫. He was from Yanshan, Hebei. His ancestors were from various cities in Shandong. He is one of the representative physicians of the Chinese-Western medical unification current (*Zhong-Xi yi huitong xuepai* 中西醫匯通學派). In 1893, he participated in—and failed—the provincial-level imperial examinations for the second time. In obedience to his father's commands, he changed his plans and began studying medicine. He broadly read the Chinese medical classics

---

1 The current text writes this as, "Feng-Zhi War 奉直戰爭," but it is usually written the other way around.

and the theories of historical physicians. Afterwards, he came into contact with Western medicine and other Western studies. Influenced by the prevailing current of ideas at the time, Mr. Zhang developed the concept of "Chinese at heart while consulting the Western" (*zhong Zhong can Xi* 衷中參西). In 1911, he accepted command of the troops garrisoned in Dezhou, becoming a medical officer and beginning his career as a practicing physician. In 1916 he founded our country's first Chinese medicine hospital in Shenyang: Lida Chinese Medicine Hospital (*Lida zhongyiyuan* 立達中醫院). In 1928, he settled in Tianjin and founded the National Medicine Correspondence School (*Guoyi hanshou xuexiao* 國醫函授學校). *Shenyang Medical Magazine, Shanghai Chinese Medicine Magazine* (*Shanghai zhongyi zazhi* 上海中醫雜誌), *Annals of the Medical World* (*Yijie chunqiu* 醫界春秋), *Triple Three Medical Journal* (*San-san yibao* 三三醫報), and *Chinese-Western Medical Magazine* (*Zhong-Xi yixue zazhi* 中西醫學雜誌)—as well as Singapore's *Medical Magazine* (*Yixue zazhi* 醫學雜誌)—all invited him to be a special contributor. In the pages of these journals, he published many particularly innovative medical articles. His most representative work, *Medicine: Chinese at Heart while Consulting the Western* (*Yixue zhong Zhong can Xi lu* 醫學衷中參西錄), in thirty sections, is a collection of a lifetime of realization through study and experience in the clinic.

Liu Jingsu "used the courtesy name Miantang 冕堂 and is a scholar-physician of Shenyang. He has long been held in high esteem in all of the provinces of the north and south. He is a doctor of the provincial capital, and his students are so numerous they almost fill the city. He has steeped himself in the medical classics for more than thirty years. In discussing theory and examining patients, he is precise and meticulous" ("A Brief Introduction to Liu Jingsu," issue 7). His writings include *Main Points of Introductory Diagnosis* (*Chubu zhenduan xue dayi* 初步診斷學大義) and *Introductory Diagnosis* (*Chubu zhenduan xue* 初步診斷學).

Shen Wenkui (1888–1958) used the courtesy name Zongzhi 宗之. His family was originally from Luanxian, Hebei. In his youth he studied medicine with the famous Shenyang physician, Zhu Kunshan 朱昆山. In 1910, he set up the Hall of Increasing Virtue (*Yishan tang* 益善堂) in Xiaonanguan where he was an expert at treating internal medicine diseases and warm disease. In 1912, he received a job offer from the *Shengjing Times* (*Shengjing shibao* 盛京時報) to open a "Medical Discussions" column. It was received very favorably and was very influential. In 1922, he was elected as the vice-president of the Fengtian Medical Research Association (*Fengtian yixue yanjiuhui* 奉天醫學研究會) (Shenyang's earliest medical association). Afterwards, he became president. After the Liberation, he became the vice-president of the Shenyang Unified Chinese-Western Medical Hospital (*Shenyang Zhong-Xi yi lianhe yiyuan* 瀋陽

中西益聯合醫院) and vice-president of the Shenyang Municipal Infectious Disease Institute (*Shenyang shi chuanranbing yuan* 瀋陽市傳染病院). In 1955, he became a member of the standing committee of the Shenyang city political consultative conference.

Ma Yinglin (1892–1969) used the courtesy names Yushu 浴書 and Shouyin 瘦吟. In his collection he had two zithers (*guqin* 古琴), one named "A Day in Autumn" and the other named "A Crystal Clear Sky." For this reason he called himself by the sobriquet "Two Zithers (*er qin* 二琴)." As a youth he studied with Liu Jingsu and Zhang Zixiang 張子鄉. He was blessed with intelligence, study broadly, and became quite learned. Apart from being an expert at medicine, he also wrote poetry, wrote excellent calligraphy, and ardently loved music. At various times he was the president of the Fengtian Medical Research Association, chair of the Shenyang National Medicine Trade Association (*Shenyang guoyi gonghui* 瀋陽國醫公會), and health maintenance consultant to the office of the general, Zhang Zuolin 張作霖. After the September 18th Incident, the Japanese puppet government of Manchuria attempted to obliterate Chinese medicine in Northeast China. In 1933, they stopped the annual Chinese medicine exam in a vain effort to cause Chinese medicine to expire on its own. In 1940, Ma Yinglin was compelled to go to Changchun Cuihua Hospital (*Changchun cuihua yiyuan* 長春翠華醫院) and struggle for superiority with Japanese medical doctors. Ma Yinglin used Chinese medicine to treat a case of purulent appendicitis. After one dose of medicine the pain diminished. After the second dose, the pain stopped. After the third dose, a Western medical examination found the patient completely cured. The Japanese had no choice but to accept that Chinese medicine had clinical efficacy. The following year they reinstated the Chinese medicine examination and invited Ma Yinglin to be a member of the Chinese medicine examination committee. Having saved Chinese medicine in the Northeast, Ma Yinglin's contributions could not go unnoticed. After the founding of the People's Republic, he was offered a position as an assistant professor and chair of the Chinese medicine teaching and research section at the Chinese Medical Science University (*Zhongguo yike daxue* 中國醫科大學). He was the first Chinese medicine physician in the country to receive the title, "assistant professor" (see, Zhang Cunti 張存悌, "The Four Famous Physicians of Old Shenyang [*Lao Shenyang sida mingyi* 老瀋陽四大名醫]," *Liaoning Chinese Medicine Magazine* [*Liaoning zhongyi zazhi* 遼寧中醫雜誌], 2004, issue 2).

11. *Guangzhou's* Chinese Medicine Magazine (Zhongyi zazhi 中醫雜誌)

In April 1926 (the fifteenth year of the Republican period), *Chinese Medicine Magazine* was founded in Guangzhou. It was edited and published by the Guangdong Chinese Medicine School (*Guangdong zhongyi zhuanmen xuexiao* 廣東中醫專門學校). This journal was printed in a 16mo format. In November 1928, it ceased publication after publishing altogether six issues. From the first issue onward, this journal set up eight columns which continued in the same style throughout its publishing run: "Monographs," "Theory," "Model Essays," "Case Histories," "Proven Formulae," "Investigations," "Miscellany," and "School News."

The Guangdong Chinese Medicine School was a high-level undergraduate professional school. Its founding was initiated by the Guangzhou-Hong Kong Crude Medicinal Warehouse and the celebrated physician Tu Gongtong 土共同. Preparations began in 1913, and in October 1916, the Chinese Medicine School Preparation Office of Guangdong and Hong Kong was formally established. Lu Naitong 盧乃潼 and Li Rongsheng 李蓉生 were elected by general acclaim as the managers of the Guangzhou Preparation Office. Wu Yaoting 伍耀庭 and Zeng Sipu 曾思普 were the Hong Kong branch Preparation Office's managers, but the provincial authorities were slow to officially register them. At the end of 1917, Lu Naitong went personally to Beijing to meet with the head of the interior ministry. Only by repeatedly suffering setbacks and exerting effort was he able to succeed. On January 15th, 1918, in the interior ministry's 198th official response, the school was approved and registered as requested. On January 27th, the 151st official response of the provincial governor of Guangdong and Guangxi was received, approving its registration and ordering the police of the provincial capital to sincerely protect it.

On September 15th, 1924, Guangdong Chinese Medicine School held its opening ceremony. In his speech, Lu Naitong, the first president of the school, said, "China's natural medicinal production is worth hundreds of millions each year. The livelihood and taxes of the common people, are mostly derived from this. If because of the decline of Chinese medicine, [the market for] Chinese medicinals also declines, the consequences will be very great. The purpose of the establishment of this school is to practice Chinese medicine in order to preserve Chinese medicinals, to understand Western medicine from the point of view of Chinese medicine, to protect our national essence, and to safeguard local products, in order to cultivate people skilled in medicine." These were

© KONINKLIJKE BRILL NV, LEIDEN, 2020 | DOI:10.1163/9789004420724_012

Mr. Lu's instructions to the students. We can also say that they were the reason the medical community of Guangdong and Hong Kong established and educational institution.

In 1955, the Guangdong Chinese Medicine School closed its doors. After more than thirty years of instruction, it had twenty-one graduating classes for a total of 571 graduates. There were also a further 322 students who studied at the school for a time but did not graduate. Altogether then, the school contributed to the training of 893 excellent Chinese medical practitioners.

12. Annals of the Medical World (Yijie chunqiu 醫界春秋)

On May 26th, 1926 (the fifteenth year of the Republican period), *Annals of the Medical World* was established in Shanghai. It was published and distributed by the Shanghai Annals of the Medical World Society (*Shanghai yijie chunqiu she* 醫界春秋社). It was published monthly in a 16mo printing format. When it was first published, the main text of the journal occupied ten pages. Over time, this increased to more than thirty pages. At the time it was established the price was fixed at four cents of a silver dollar (*dayang sifen* 大洋四分). Afterwards, the price was repeatedly adjusted. In March 1937, the journal ceased publication having published altogether 123 issues.

The purpose of this journal was to allow the Chinese medical community to learn from one another by exchanging views. Regarding content, it strove "to judge the quality without regard to whether it is Chinese or Western," "to distinguish truth and falsehood while not esteeming on vilification," and "to be devoted to truth and place no value on empty talk." In seeking contributions, the requirements were that the article "is relevant to the affairs of Chinese or Western medicine, reaches a firm conclusion on the basis of facts, or brings together theories and principles so that they mutually corroborate each other" ("Introduction [*Fakanci* 發刊詞]"). This journal was founded against the background of a society in which Chinese and Western medicine were contending with one another. Its purpose was to create a center for public discourse within the medical community. They hoped to establish provide fair guidance for the medical community's discussions by means of deliberation within that community.

Most of the contributors to the journal were members of the Annals of the Medical World Society. The journal was edited by the Society, but in reality the primary editorial work was primarily handled by the chair of the Society, Zhang Zanchen 張贊臣. From the thirty-seventh issue onward, the journal clearly stated that Zhang Zanchen was the chief editor. Among the several tens of famous Chinese medical physicians who wrote for the journal were Zhang Taiyan 章太炎, Meng Sou 矇叟, Bao Shisheng 包識生, Yun Tieqiao 惲鐵樵, Lu Pusheng 陸普笙, Lu Shi'e 陸士諤, Xie Liheng 謝利恆, and Zhu Weiju 祝味菊.

The editor-in-chief, Zhang Zanchen (1904–1993) was from Wujin, Jiangsu. He used the courtesy name Jixun 繼勛 and later in life the sobriquets "Old Man Teapot (*Husou* 壺叟)" and "the Old Man of Rong Lake (*Ronghu laoren* 蓉湖老人)." Mr. Zhang was born in a family of hereditary physicians. His grandfather

© KONINKLIJKE BRILL NV, LEIDEN, 2020 | DOI:10.1163/9789004420724_013

Ming 銘 and his father Boxi 伯熙 were both famous physicians of Wujin, Jiangsu, who were particularly skilled in internal medicine, ailments of the skin, and illnesses of the throat. In his youth, Zhang Zanchen practiced medicine with his father, laying a solid foundation of medical theory and clinical skills. At sixteen he accompanied his father to Shanghai and entered the Shanghai Chinese Medicine School (*Shanghai zhongyi zhuanmen xuexiao* 上海中醫專門學校). Later, he enrolled in the Shanghai Chinese Medicine University (*Shanghai zhongyi daxue* 上海中醫大學) and continued to pursue advanced studies. In 1926, he graduated with honors (the program lasted six years). Afterwards he studied further with the famous Shanghai physicians Xie Liheng, Cao Yingfu 曹 穎甫, and Bao Shisheng. He possessed both a deep family tradition of medical study and an excellent formal education. After graduating, he practiced medicine in Shanghai and mastered the departments of internal medicine, skin diseases, gynecology, pediatrics, and EENT. He was particularly skilled in treating skin and throat diseases. In addition to his clinical work, he also worked as a teacher for the Chinese Medical School, actively participated in Chinese medical public welfare activities, energetically founded Chinese medical organizations, and participated in association activities. Apart from supporting the Annals of the Medical World Society and acting as editor-in-chief for *Annals of the Medical World* magazine, he also founded or participated in the founding of the Shanghai National Medicine Institute (*Shanghai guoyi jiangxisuo* 上海國 醫講習所), the Chinese Medical Research Institute (*Zhongguo yiyao yanjiusuo* 中國醫藥研究所), the Shanghai Chinese Medicine School, and the Shanghai Municipal Chinese Physician's Research Association (*Shanghai shi zhongyi shi yanjiuhui* 上海市中醫師研究會). He was the editor-in-chief of the *Journal of Elementary Medical Knowledge* (*Yiyao changshi bao* 醫藥常識報) and *Annals of the Medical World*. He became a particularly influential theorist, clinician, and publisher with in the Chinese medical community of the Republican period. After 1949, he emphasized his work on Chinese medical treatment of the ears, nose, and throat. In 1956 he participated in the establishment of the Shanghai Chinese Medical Literature Institute (*Shanghai zhongyi wenxian guan* 上海中醫文獻館). He later became the Institute's vice-president. He was a professor and chair of the ears, nose, and throat teaching and research group at the Shanghai College of Chinese Medicine (*Shanghai zhongyi xueyuan* 上海中醫學院) and became one of the founders of the China Chinese Medical ENT Association. He was also honorary chair of that association, vice-chair of the Shanghai Municipal Chinese Medical Association (*Shanghai shi zhongyi xuehui* 上海市中醫學會), and a consultant for the Shanghai College of Chinese Medicine's affiliate, Shuguang Hospital (*Shuguang yiyuan* 曙光醫院).

13. Chinese Medical Monthly (Zhongguo yixue yuekan 中國醫學月刊)

On October 1st, 1928 (the seventeenth year of the Republican period), *Chinese Medical Monthly* was founded in Shanghai. Lu Yuanlei 陸淵雷 was editor-in-chief and the Chinese Medical Monthly Society were the editors. It was published monthly, at first on the first day of every month. After the sixth issue was published, the publishing date changed to the tenth of every month. The eleventh issue was published in April 1930, eleven issues are currently extant (Shanghai Medical Museum [*Shanghai yiyaoxue bowuguan* 上海醫藥學博物館] holds copies of issues one through ten and the Chinese Academy of Chinese Medical Science [*Zhongguo zhongyi kexueyuan* 中國中醫科學院] holds a copy of issue eleven. Copies of issue 12 and later issues have yet to be found.).

Lu Yuanlei (1894–1955) was named Pengnian 彭年 and was from Chuansha district, Shanghai (now the Pudong New District). In 1912 he entered Jiangsu Province Number One Teacher's School (*Jiangsu sheng diyi shifan daxue* 江蘇省第一師範大學). He studied the Confucian classics and philology with the great master of textual studies (*puxue* 樸學), Yao Mengxun 姚孟醺. In 1925, Yun Tieqiao 惲鐵樵 founded the Medical Correspondence School (*Yixue hanshou xuexiao* 醫學函授學校), and Lu Yuanlei formally became his student and assisted in running the school. He later also took the great classical scholar Mr. Zhang Taiyan 章太炎 as his teacher for classical Chinese and fundamentals of Chinese medicine. In 1928, together with Xu Hengzhi 徐衡之 and Zhang Cigong 章次公, he founded the Shanghai National Medicine College (*Shanghai guoyi xueyuan* 上海國醫學院).

Lu Yuanlei is one of the modern representatives of the Chinese-Western medical unification current (*Zhong-Xi yi huitong xuepai* 中西醫匯通學派). Along with emphasizing the need to develop Chinese medicine, he actively borrowed from Western studies. Around 1932, he became a member of the Central National Medicine Institute's Scholarly Reform Committee (*Zhongyang guoyi guan xueshu zhengli weiyuanhui* 中央國醫館學術整理委員會). In 1934, he founded *Chinese Medicine's New Life* (*Zhongyi xin shengming* 中醫新生命) and became its editor-in-chief. After the founding of the People's Republic, Lu Yuanlei at various times was vice-chair of the Shanghai Municipal Medical Science Research Committee (*Shanghai shi yikexue yanjiu weiyuanhui* 上海市醫科學研究委員會), chair of the Shanghai Municipal Chinese Medicine Association (*Shanghai shi zhongyi xuehui* 上海市中醫學會), Chinese medicine consultant to the Shanghai Municipal Department of Public Health

© KONINKLIJKE BRILL NV, LEIDEN, 2020 | DOI:10.1163/9789004420724_014

(*Shanghai shi weishengju* 上海市衛生局), and director of the Shanghai Chinese Medicine Clinic (*Shanghai zhongyi menzhensuo* 上海中醫門診所). He was deeply involved in clinical practice and teaching for a long time. In his studies, he emphasized classical formulae as well as assimilating new knowledge. His writings are particularly abundant, including *A Modern Explanation of the Treatise on Cold Damage* (*Shanghan lun jinshi* 傷寒論今釋), *A Modern Explanation of Essentials of the Golden Coffer* (*Jingui yaolue jinshi* 金匱要略今釋), *Mr. Lu's Collected Writings* (*Lu shi jilun* 陸氏集論), *An Explanation of the Chinese Medical Physiology Terminology* (*Zhongyi shengli shuyu jie* 中醫生理術語解), *An Explanation of Chinese Medical Pathology Terminology* (*Zhongyi bingli shuyu jie* 中醫病理術語解), *Essentials of Epidemic Disease* (*Liuxing bing xuzhi* 流行病須知), and *An Outline of the Treatise on Cold Damage* (*Shanghan lun gaiyao* 傷寒論概要).

This journal never settled on a fixed style for either its cover or its columns. The first through fifth issues used the simple style of using an inspirational quote on the journal's cover. Afterwards, due to procrastination on all fronts and personnel changes, the sixth issue was delayed by four months, only coming out on July 10th of the following year. After redesign, the new cover used the English words, "China Medical Journal." The content of the covers for the seventh through ninth issues was more substantial, having been designed by an art designer, and bore the slogan "The Ten Thousand Illnesses are Restored to Health (*wanbing huichun* 萬病回春)." However, the cover of the tenth issue returned to a simple form again. The person writing the inscription for the cover also changed repeatedly. For the first, second, and seventh issues, Bai Longjiu 白龍久 wrote it. For the third issue, Wang Zheng 王正, a founding member of the Communist Party was invited to write it. The inscription for the fourth and fifth issues were written by Mr. Zhang Taiyan himself. The inscriptions for the eighth and ninth issues were written by the painter and calligrapher Meng Shouzhi 蒙壽芝. The tenth and eleventh issues used block print.

14. Apricot Grove Medical Monthly (Xinglin yixue yuebao 杏林醫學月報)

In January 1929 (the eighteenth year of the Republican period), the *Apricot Grove Medical Monthly* was founded in Guangzhou. It was edited, published, and distributed by the Apricot Grove Medical Monthly Society (*Xinglin yixue yuebao she* 杏林醫學月報社). One issue was released each month and twelve issues were released each year—with the exception of February and December of 1929, in which no issue was published for unknown reasons. Altogether, 101 issues were published. The journal ceased publication in July 1937. More than one thousand copies of each issue were published. For Republican-period Guangzhou, it is one of the longest-running and most uninterrupted medical publications and has the largest number of issues and most complete publishing run still extant. More than two hundred writers contributed to the journal, and more than 1400 articles were published altogether. The content included medical theory, medical cases, medical discussions, and medical affairs.

The editors-in-chief were Zhang Jieping 張階平 and Jiang Kun 江堃. Zhang Jieping (1906–1985) was from Shunde, Guangdong. He was a graduate of Guangdong Chinese Medicine School (*Guangdong zhongyi zhuanmen xuexiao* 廣東中醫專門學校) and was one of the founders of the Guangdong Chinese Medicine Hospital (*Guangdong zhongyiyuan* 廣東中醫院). He was a professor at Guangdong Chinese Medicine School, an assistant professor at Guangzhou Chinese Medicine College (*Guangzhou zhongyi xueyuan* 廣州中醫學院), and an attending internal medicine physician at the Guangdong Provincial Chinese Medical Hospital (*Guangdong sheng zhongyiyuan* 廣東省中醫院). In 1962 and 1978 he was awarded the title "Guangdong Province Senior Physician of Chinese Medicine." Throughout his life, Zhang practiced Chinese medicine in the clinic, wrote books and propounded arguments, and passed on the torch of the learning of Qibo and the Yellow Emperor.

Apricot Grove Medical Monthly was published in the 1920s and '30s. At that time Chinese medicine was undergoing a period of devastation and suppression. Even though things were like this, this journal still persevered in publishing for more than eight years. It fought for the strengthening of Chinese medicine, gave impetus to the development of Chinese medicine, and disseminated Chinese medical knowledge. It fought for Chinese medicine's right to exist and provided it with a firm stage from which to speak. It became a tactically important position for the scholarship and public discussion of Chinese medical community of Republican period Guangdong.

© KONINKLIJKE BRILL NV, LEIDEN, 2020 | DOI:10.1163/9789004420724_015

15. Guangdong Medical Monthly (Guangdong yiyao yuebao 廣東醫藥月報)

In the January 1929 (the eighteenth year of the Republican period), *Guangdong Medical Monthly* was founded in Guangdong by the Guangdong New Chinese Medicine Association (*Guangdong xin zhongyi xuehui* 廣東新中醫學會). The publicity committee of the Guangdong New Chinese Medicine Association edited and distributed it. This journal was published monthly for a total of nine issues. Among these, the third and fourth issues were the first and second parts of a "Special Issue on Medical Trends (*Yichao tekan hao* 醫潮特刊號)." The seventh issue was a "Special Issue on the Chinese Teaching Materials Editorial Conference (*Zhongyi jiaocai bianji huiyi zhuanhao* 中醫教材編輯會議專號)."

The Guangdong New Chinese Medicine Association's mission was to carry forward traditional Chinese culture, hasten the development of Chinese medicine, strengthen the interaction and communication between Chinese and Western medicine, and promote the cause of human health. According to this journal's "Introduction (*Fakanci* 發刊詞)" (in the inaugural issue), there were three purposes for founding the journal: first, preserving Chinese knowledge of medicine and hygiene, as well as enhancing its ongoing organization and innovation; second, researching the most recent knowledge of medicine and hygiene from foreign countries in order to remedy our medicine's inadequacies while making this journal a window on Chinese medicine for the rest of the world and strengthening communication between Chinese and Western medicine; and third, to advance the cause of aiding human health by introducing basic information about medicine and hygiene and disseminating medical knowledge.

© KONINKLIJKE BRILL NV, LEIDEN, 2020 | DOI:10.1163/9789004420724_016

16. Chinese Medical World (Zhongyi shijie 中醫世界)

In June 1929 (the eighteenth year of the Republican period), *Chinese Medical World* was founded in Shanghai. It was published by Chinese Medicine Press (*Zhongyi shuju* 中醫書局), who invited Qin Bowei 秦伯未 and Fang Gongbo 方公溥 to be editors-in-chief. They also invited more than twenty nationally famous people—including Zhang Taiyan 章太炎 and Xia Yingtang 夏應堂—to be special contributors. This journal was published in a 32mo publishing format. This journal was originally planned as a bimonthly publication with six issues per year as one volume. The first and fourth issues of each volume were to be special issues. Later on this was modified in the course of the work. In order to increase reader interest, the journal was changed to a monthly publication for the third and fourth volumes. In order to increase the length of the journal, the journal became a seasonal publication in the fifth and sixth volumes. In order to make the information more timely, from the seventh volume onward, the journal returned to monthly publication. In order to improve its reputation, from the eight year onward, *Chinese Medical World* adhered strictly to publishing issues on schedule and steadily matured and improved. Starting with volume 5, the table of contents began displaying page numbers. Beginning with volume 9, the journal was divided into sections and the editorial committee invited Qiu Zhizhong 邱治中, Sheng Xinru 盛心如, and Jiang Wenfang 蔣文芳 to join the committee. They then further invited twenty more people—including Tang Jishan 唐吉山 and Yu Qishan 俞岐山—to be special contributors. There was also a significant change to the cover of the journal. From volume 10 onward, this journal was published together with *The Record of Chinese Medical Guidance* (*Zhongyi zhidao lu* 中醫指導錄), with that journal appended to the end of this one (see the synopsis of *The Record of Chinese Medical Guidance*). *Chinese Medical World* was published through August 1937, and then ceased publication (volume 12, issue 5, was delayed until October of that year due to the August 13th Incident). The journal published a total of twelve volumes and sixty-seven issues. The journal was forced to halt publication because of the Japanese invasion of China. "An Urgent Statement from this Society" in volume 12, issue 5, states "On 'August 13th' the Japanese attack on Shanghai commenced. Communications were obstructed and all services halted. This Society and like-minded people engaged in providing emergency relief. The Society's activities were then brought to a close. Two months have passed, but it is still difficult to resume them. Apart from striving to publish

© KONINKLIJKE BRILL NV, LEIDEN, 2020 | DOI:10.1163/9789004420724_017

this issue, when the hostilities have abated, we will make up for our current inability. All correspondence has been saved and is waiting until we have time to respond."

Qin Bowei (1901–1970) was named Zhiji 之濟 and used the sobriquet Qianzhai 謙齋. He was from Shanghai county, Jiangsu (modern Minhang district, Shanghai). He was an outstanding physician of the times. He was born in a family of scholar-physicians and from his youth loved classical literature and medical texts. He first studied medicine with Cao Yingfu 曹穎甫. In 1919 he entered the Shanghai Chinese Medical School (*Shanghai zhongyi zhuanmen xuexiao* 上海中醫專門學校) and assiduously studied Chinese medicine under Ding Ganren 丁甘仁. In 1923, after graduating, he practiced clinical Chinese medicine, taught, and published. He founded the National Medicine Press (*Guoyi shuju* 國醫書局) (Chinese Medicine Press) and taught at the Shanghai National Medicine College (*Shanghai guoyi xueyuan* 上海國醫學院) and the New Chinese Medicine College (*Xin zhongyi xueyuan* 新中醫學院). After the founding of the People's Republic, he was a Chinese medicine consultant for the department of public health and was chosen as the vice-president of the Chinese Medicine Association (*Zhonghua yixuehui* 中華醫學會). His publications include *A Simple Explanation of the Essentials of the Inner Classic* (*Neijing zhiyao qianjie* 內經知要淺解), *Essentials of Chinese Clinical Practice* (*Zhongyi linzheng beiyao* 中醫臨證備要), and *Qianzhai's Medical Lectures* (*Qianzhai yixue jianggao* 謙齋醫學講稿). He energetically participated in the propagation of Chinese medical culture. With his simple and unpretentious scholarly character, he made an important contribution to the rescuing of Chinese medicine and the development of the interchange of Chinese medical knowledge.

17. Self-Strengthening Medical Monthly (Ziqiang yixue yuekan 自強醫學月刊) (Self-Strengthening Medical Journal [Ziqiang yikan 自強醫刊])

In October 1929 (the eighteenth year of the Republican period), *Self-Strengthening Medical Monthly* was founded in Shanghai. Zhu Weiju 祝味菊, Lu Yuanlei 陸淵雷, Xu Hengzhi 徐衡之, and Liu Sigao 劉泗橋 together acted as editors-in-chief. In October 1931, it ceased publication, having published twenty issues altogether. Starting with the seventh issue, the title on the cover was changed to *"Self-Strengthening Medical Journal"* (the fifteenth and sixteenth issues were published as a combined issue). The calligraphy on the journal's cover was written by Zhang Bingllin 章炳麟, Chen Jiayou 陳嘉佑, Shi Jinmo 施今墨, and Wang Zhen 王震. Issues one through six lacked clearly distinguished columns. Beginning with issue 7, there were improvements. The cover and layout were adjusted, and the following specialized columns were established: "Preface," "Criticism," "Theory," and "Reader's Letters." They also began publishing longer articles in installments.

Zhu Weiju (1884–1951) was also known by the sobriquet, "Master of the High Places, Unbent by Frost (*Aoshuang Xuanzhu* 傲霜軒主)."[1] His ancestral home was in Shanyin (in modern Shaoxing, Zhejiang), but he was born in Chengdu, Sichuan. His forebears were hereditary physicians. As a youth he worked with his uncle, managing the salt business in Chengdu. His uncle asked the old scholar, Liu Yusheng 劉雨笙 to teach Zhu the medical classics. He also studied at a military medical school. Later on, he studied with the Japanese teacher, Ishida, and traveled to Japan to study Western medicine. After returning to China, he took a position at the hospital the Sichuan provincial government had established in Chengdu and had a good medical reputation. After 1917, he moved to Shanghai where he taught successively at the Shanghai Chinese Medicine School (*Shanghai zhongyi zhuanmen xuexiao* 上海中醫專門學校) and the China Medical College (*Zhongguo yixueyuan* 中國醫學院), and also became president of the New China Medical Research Institute (*Xinzhongguo yixue yanjiuyuan* 新中國醫學研究院). In 1927, with Xu Xiaofu 徐小圃 and others, began establishing Jinghe Medical Science University (*Jinghe yike daxue* 景和醫科大學). In 1937, with the Western medical physicians, Mei Zhuosheng 梅卓生 and Lan Na 蘭納, set up a combined Chinese and Western medical clinic. After Zhu Weiju came to Shanghai, he often discussed medical theory

---

1 Xuanzhu 軒主 is also one of the titles of the Yellow Emperor.

© KONINKLIJKE BRILL NV, LEIDEN, 2020 | DOI:10.1163/9789004420724_018

with the famous Shanghai physicians, Xu Xiangren 徐相任, Lu Yuanlei, and Zhang Cigong 章次公. He emphasized the need for Chinese medical reform, holding that "If we wish to propagate the ancient principles, we must merge them with modern knowledge."

Lu Yuanlei (1894–1955) was named Pengnian 彭年 and was from Chuansha district, Shanghai (now the Pudong New District). In 1912 he entered Jiangsu Province Number One Teacher's School (*Jiangsu sheng diyi shifan daxue* 江蘇省第一師範大學). He studied the Confucian classics and philology with the great master of textual studies (*puxue* 樸學), Yao Mengxun 姚孟醺. In 1925, Yun Tieqiao 惲鐵樵 founded the Medical Correspondence School (*Yixue hanshou xuexiao* 醫學函授學校), and Lu Yuanlei formally became his student and assisted in running the school. He later also took the great classical scholar Mr. Zhang Taiyan 章太炎 as his teacher for classical Chinese and fundamentals of Chinese medicine. In 1928, together with Xu Hengzhi and Zhang Cigong, he founded the Shanghai National Medicine College (*Shanghai guoyi xueyuan* 上海國醫學院). Lu Yuanlei is one of the modern representatives of the Chinese-Western medical unification current (*Zhong-Xi yi huitong xuepai* 中西醫匯通學派). Along with emphasizing the need to develop Chinese medicine, he actively borrowed from Western studies. Around 1932, he became a member of the Central National Medicine Institute's Scholarly Reform Committee (*Zhongyang guoyi guan xueshu zhengli weiyuanhui* 中央國醫館學術整理委員會). In 1934, he founded *Chinese Medicine's New Life* (*Zhongyi xinshengming* 中醫新生命) and became its editor-in-chief. After the founding of the People's Republic, Lu Yuanlei at various times was vice-chair of the Shanghai Municipal Medical Science Research Committee (*Shanghai shi yikexue yanjiu weiyuanhui* 上海市醫科學研究委員會), chair of the Shanghai Municipal Chinese Medicine Association (*Shanghai shi zhongyi xuehui* 上海市中醫學會), Chinese medicine consultant to the Shanghai Municipal Department of Public Health (*Shanghai shi weishengju* 上海市衛生局), and director of the Shanghai Chinese Medicine Clinic (*Shanghai zhongyi menzhensuo* 上海中醫門診所). He was deeply involved in clinical practice and teaching for a long time. In his studies, he emphasized classical formulae as well as assimilating new knowledge. His writings are particularly abundant, including *A Modern Explanation of the Treatise on Cold Damage* (*Shanghan lun jinshi* 傷寒論今釋), *A Modern Explanation of Essentials of the Golden Coffer* (*Jingui yaolue jinshi* 金匱要略今釋), *Mr. Lu's Collected Writings* (*Lu shi jilun* 陸氏集論), *An Explanation of the Chinese Medical Physiology Terminology* (*Zhongyi shengli shuyu jie* 中醫生理術語解), *An Explanation of Chinese Medical Pathology Terminology* (*Zhongyi bingli shuyu jie* 中醫病理術語解), *Essentials of Epidemic Disease* (*Liuxing bing xuzhi* 流行病須知), and *An Outline of the Treatise on Cold Damage* (*Shanghan lun gaiyao* 傷寒論概要).

Xu Hengzhi (1903–1968) was from Changzhou, Jiangsu. In 1922, he graduated from the Shanghai Chinese Medicine School. Afterwards, he studied and practiced with Yun Tieqiao and also taught at Tieqiao's correspondence school. At the same time, he discussed medical problems with Mr. Zhang Taiyan. In 1928, he founded the Shanghai National Medicine College with Lu Yuanlei and Zhang Cigong. He also became a member of the National Chinese Medicine Federation (*Quanguo zhongyi lianhehui* 全國中醫聯合會) and began the establishment of the Central National Medicine Institute (*Zhongyang guoyi guan* 中央國醫館), in which he became an honorary board member and director of the Shanghai branch. He was also chair of the Chinese medicine section of the Shanghai Red Cross Hospital. After this he practiced medicine for many years in Shanghai and Changzhou, successfully treating many difficult cases.

Liu Sigao (1897–1930) was from Zhenhai, Zhejiang. As a child he was very clever. Later, he studied Chinese medicine intensively. Having completed his studies, he practiced medicine on his own in Shanghai. His skills were masterful. He also taught at the Shanghai National Medicine College and translated and published *Imperial Chinese Medicine* (*Kōkan igaku* 皇漢醫學) by the famous Japanese doctor of Chinese medicine, Yumoto Kyūshin 湯本求真. Liu made a definite contribution to the development of modern Chinese medicine.

18. The Record of Chinese Medical Guidance (Zhongyi zhidao lu 中醫指導錄)

In June 1930 (the nineteenth year of the Republican period), *The Record of Chinese Medical Guidance* was founded in Shanghai. It was a monthly publication: one issue each month, one volume every year. It was published in a 32mo printing format and each issue was approximately 30 pages long. At the time it ceased publication, in May, 1936, it had published altogether six volumes and seventy-two issues. It had not missed publication of a single issue for those six years. According to a "Notice (*Qishi* 啓事)" in volume 6, issue 72, this journal was henceforth to be published together with *Chinese Medical World* (*Zhongyi shijie* 中醫世界) (edited by Qin Bowei 秦伯未 and Fang Gongpu 方公溥).

The cover of this journal at first was inscribed "Managed by Qin Bowei 秦伯未 and Xu Banlong 需半龍, Edited by the Chinese Medical Guidance Society." After volume 1, issue 7, it began to say merely "Edited by the Chinese Medical Guidance Society" or "Edited by the Chinese Medical Guidance Society (Managed by Qin Bowei)." It did not again include Mr. Xu's name. "Seventh Announcement by this Society [*Benshe qishi qi* 本社啟事七]," in volume 2, issue 21, states "Although responsibility for the Society's activities is divided among all members, the person who oversees their success is Bowei alone." From this one can see that when this journal began Qin Bowei and Xu Banlong together acted as editors-in-chief, but afterwards, Xu Banlong withdrew, leaving Qin Bowei alone as the editor-in-chief.

Qin Bowei (1901–1970) was named Zhiji 之濟 and used the sobriquet Qianzhai 謙齋. He was from Shanghai county, Jiangsu (modern Minhang district, Shanghai). He was born to a family of hereditary physicians. His grandfather Diqiao 笛樵, his father Yangqi 錫棋, and his uncle Yangtian 錫田 were all well-versed in medicine and traditional scholarship. In 1919, Qin Bowei entered Ding Ganren's 丁甘仁 Shanghai Chinese Medicine School (*Shanghai zhongyi zhuanmen xuexiao* 上海中醫專門學校). He was a student of the school's third class, and was schoolmates with Cheng Menxue 程門雪 and Zhang Cigong 章次公. After graduating, he took a post as a teacher at Shanghai Chinese Medicine School and the Shanghai Chinese Medicine College. He founded the National Medicine Press (*Guoyi shuju* 國醫書局) (the Chinese Medicine Press [*Zhongyi shuju* 中醫書局]) and the Chinese Medicine Guidance Society. Apart from publishing medical texts, the Chinese Medicine Press was also responsible for publishing two medical magazines, *Chinese Medical World* and *Family Medical Magazine* (*Jiating yixue zazhi* 家庭醫學雜誌). Both were edited by Qin

© KONINKLIJKE BRILL NV, LEIDEN, 2020 | DOI:10.1163/9789004420724_019

Bowei and Fang Gongpu 方公溥. After the founding of the People's Republic, Qin Bowei was a Chinese medicine consultant for the department of public health, vice-president of the Chinese Medicine Association (*Zhonghua yixue-hui* 中華醫學會), and dean of studies at Beijing College of Chinese Medicine (*Beijing zhongyi xueyuan* 北京中醫學院). The *Sea of Words'* (*Cihai* 辭海), "Qin Bowei" entry, evaluates him in this way: "He had many attainments in the study of Chinese medicine. He was well-versed in Chinese medical theory and also skilled in Chinese medical theory, poetry, and calligraphy." He founded many Chinese medical organizations, edited many types of Chinese medical maga-zine, authored and published a great deal of Chinese medical teaching mate-rial and other books. He made many lasting contributions to the cultivation of skilled Chinese medical physicians and the development of Chinese medicine.

Xu Banlong (1898–1939) was also named Guanzeng 觀曾 and used the cour-tesy name Yufu 畬孚. He was Wujiang, Jiangsu. He started studying under Jin Tianhe 金天翮 and continued studying medicine with his uncle Chen Zhongwei 陳仲威. Later, he graduated from Shanghai Chinese Medical School. In the clinic he was particularly adept with skin diseases. He was chair of the department of skin diseases at the Shanghai Guangyi Hospital (*Shanghai guangyi yiyuan* 上海廣益醫院) and enjoyed a moment of fleeting fame. In 1927, together with Qin Bowei, he established the Shanghai Chinese Medicine College (Shanghai *Zhongguo yixueyuan* 上海中國醫學院) and was a teacher at that school. His writings include *An Outline of Chinese Skin Diseases* (*Zhongguo waikexue dagang* 中國外科學大綱), *The Treatment of Sores* (*Yangkexue* 瘍科學), *The Treatment of Throat Diseases* (*Houkexue* 喉科學), *Unlocking the Secrets of Medicinal Vines* (*Yaolian qimi* 藥薟啓秘), *An Overview of Internal Medicine* (*Neike gaiyao* 內科概要), and *Chinese Medicinal Formulas* (*Zhongguo fangji xue* 中國方劑學).

The Record of Chinese Medical Guidance was the only periodical published by the Chinese Medical Guidance Society that Qin Bowei founded. Regarding the Chinese Medical Guidance Society, *The Record of Chinese Medical Guid-ance* publicized it, saying, "A survey of the activities of the Chinese Medical Guidance Society: the medical section introduces new Chinese medical pub-lications and points out the way to study medicine; the social section receives medical consultations and resolves difficult cases; the research section man-ages a Chinese medical night school and supports wide-ranging research" (volume 1, issue 1).

19. *Hong Kong's* National Medicine Magazine (Guoyi zazhi 國醫雜誌)

In autumn of 1930 (the nineteenth year of the Republican period), *National Medicine Magazine* was founded by You Lie 尤列 and others in Hong Kong. It was edited by He Peiyu 何佩瑜, Li Qinshi 黎琴石, and Liao Mengpei 廖孟培 and published by the Hong Kong Chinese National Medicine Association (*Xianggang Zhonghua guoyi xuehui* 香港中華國醫學會). The publishing dates are listed as Spring, Summer, Autumn, and Winter. The precise publication dates are not specified. The journal's name on the first through twenty-first issues as well as the commemorative special issue are written in You Lie's hand. For the twenty-second issue, Jiao Yitang 焦易堂 wrote the title. Including the commemorative special issue published in February, 1936, a total of twenty-three issues were published. *The Compilation of Chinese Medicine Periodicals from the Late Qing and Republican Periods* (*Zhongguo jindai zhongyiyao qikan huibian* 中國近代中醫藥期刊彙編) lacks issues five through eight. We have inquired everywhere and are unable to find them. This journal's purpose was to "develop Chinese medicine, organize that which we already have, and promote new knowledge. Within the scope of medicine we do not publish summaries in foreign script." Each issue opened with the columns "A Sponsor's Portrait," "The Main Point of this Magazine," and "Staff Member's Names and Curriculum Vitae." "Hong Kong Chinese Medicine at a Glance" was appended to the end of each issue. The journal's content was abundant and its form variable.

You Lie (1866–1936) used the courtesy name Lingji 令季, another courtesy name Shaowan 少紈, the sobriquets Xiaoyuan 小園 and Wuxing Lizi 吳型李子, and later in life the sobriquet Bohua Daoren 鉢華道人. He was from Shunde, Guangdong. At the age of seventeen he joined the anti-Qing secret society Hongmen 洪門. At twenty-two he enrolled in the Guangzhou Mathematics Institute (*Guangzhou suanxue guan* 廣州算學館) and came to know Sun Yat-sen (Sun Zhongshan 孫中山) and Zheng Shiliang 鄭士良. Together with Sun Yat-sen, Yang Heling 楊鶴齡, and Chen Shaobai 陳少白, he advocated for the overthrow of the Qing and revolution. People of the time referred to You, Sun, Yang, and Chen as "the four great bandits (*si dakou* 四大寇)." In 1895 he participated in the formation of the Hong Kong Revive China Society (*Xingzhong hui* 興中會). He helped plan and prepare for the revolution in Guangzhou and participated in the Huizhou 惠州 uprising. In 1900 he moved to Japan. He had been selected as the president of the Zhonghe Hall (*Zhonghe tang* 中和堂).

© KONINKLIJKE BRILL NV, LEIDEN, 2020 | DOI:10.1163/9789004420724_020

The following year he moved to Nanyang. In each place he formed branch associations of the Zhonghe Hall. In order to maintain communication with the workers and small shop-owners among the overseas Chinese community, he established newspaper, *Seeking the South Daily*, in Singapore to spread revolutionary thought. When the United League of China (*Tongmeng hui* 同盟會) was established, the Zhonghe Hall joined it. After the 1911 Revolution, he opposed Yuan Shikai 袁世凱 proclamation of himself as emperor and formed the Army to Save the World (*Jiushi jun* 救世軍)[1] and engaged in the "Denouncing Yuan Shikai Movement (*tao Yuan huodong* 討袁活動)." In 1921, he became a consultant for Sun Yat-sen on military affairs and security. Afterwards he divorced himself from government affairs and resided in Hong Kong, establishing and giving lectures at the Huangjue Academy (*Huangjue shuyuan* 皇覺書院), making his living as a teacher of children. In 1936, in spite of illness, he came to the capital in person to explain his plan to save the country. Shortly thereafter he died from his illness in Nanjing. His writings include *An Easy Explanation of the Four Books by Chapter and Phrase* (*Sishu zhangju yijie* 四書章句易解) and *New Cases for the Four Books* (*Sishu xin'an* 四書新案).

---

1 The Chinese characters are the same used in the translation of the Salvation Army's name but should not be confused with it.

20. Straight Talk from the Medical World (Yilin yi'e 醫林一谔)

In January 1931 (the twentieth year of the Republican period), *Straight Talk from the Medical World* was founded in Guangzhou. It was one of the more long-running and influential of the Republican-period medical periodicals. At first, Li Zhongshou 李仲守 and Chen Yiyi 陳亦毅 acted as editors-in-chief together. In January 1932, Chen Yiyi left to take a post at a hospital and resigned from the editorial work. From that point until the journal cease publication, Li Zhongshou alone was editor-in-chief. This journal was published by the "Lingnan Straight Talk from the Medical World Society (*Lingnan yilin yikui* 嶺南醫林一諤社)." Each month there was one number (issue). In May-June 1935, the journal ceased publication. Altogether it published five volumes and fifty-four issues. Apart from its regular publication, this journal also published bound multi-issue editions as well. Usually, it was a half-year (six issues) published as one book.

Li Zhongshou (1909–1964) was from Shunde, Guangdong. He was born to a family of hereditary Chinese physicians. In 1926 he enrolled in the Guangdong Chinese Medicine Specialized Training School (*Guangdong zhongyi zhuanke xuexiao* 廣東中醫專科學校) and achieved outstanding results. In 1931, he graduated but remained at the school as a teacher. He had previously edited the *Journal of Medicine* (*Yiyao xuebao* 醫藥學報). Since that journal had ceased publication, he established the magazine, *Straight Talk from the World of Medicine* and put his whole effort into editing and publishing the journal. In 1958, he accepted an invitation to work at Guangzhou College of Chinese Medicine (*Guangzhou zhongyi xueyuan* 廣州中醫學院). He was also the chair of the Internal Medicine Association of the Guangdong branch of the Chinese Medicine Association (*Zhongyi xuehui* 中醫學會), a consultant for the Internal Medicine Association of the All-China Chinese Medicine Association (*Zhonghua quanguo zhongyi xuehui* 中華全國中醫學會), a member of the academic committee of Guangzhou College of Chinese Medicine, and a member of the Fifth Guangdong Provincial Political Consultative Conference. He was one of Guangdong Province's famous senior Chinese medical physicians. His publications were quite abundant—more than twenty items, including *Digging into Raw Herbal Medicinals* (*Sheng caoyao juefa* 生草藥掘發) and *Chance Conversations on Medicine Revised* (*Yiyu oulu* 醫餘偶錄).

© KONINKLIJKE BRILL NV, LEIDEN, 2020 | DOI:10.1163/9789004420724_021

21. Shenzhou National Medicine Journal (Shenzhou guoyi xuebao 神州國醫學報)

In January 1932 (the twenty-first year of the Republican period), *Shenzhou National Medicine Journal* was founded in Shanghai. It was edited and published by the Editorial Committee of the Shenzhou National Medicine Association (*Shenzhou guoyi xuehui* 神州國醫學會). It was printed newspaper-style on a full sheet. At first it was issued on the fifteenth of every month, but due to the fighting going on, it was sometimes delayed or only issued once every two months or every season. It survived for six years, ceasing publication in July 1937, having published a total of fifty-eight issues. Cheng Diren 程迪仁 was the director of this journal. Committee members included Wu Quji 吳去疾, Qin Shanzheng 秦善徵, Jin Changkang 金長康, and Zhang Zhiying 張志英. In actuality, starting with volume 1, issue 3, the work of editing was primarily handled by Wu Quji. The famous physician and member of the Shenzhou National Medicine Association Standing Committee, Gu Weichuan 顧渭川 wrote the journal title in his calligraphy. The Shenzhou National Medicine Association was the previous Shenzhou Medical Trade Association (*Shenzhou yiyao zonghui* 神州醫藥總會), which had changed its name in 1931. Previously, the Trade Association had published the *Shenzhou Medical Journal* (*Shenzhou yiyao xuebao* 神州醫藥學報) among other publications.

The fate of this journal was tightly tied to that of the Shenzhou National Medicine Association. Its history was full of ups and downs. First (1929), owing to the Nationalist government edict, "medicine and pharmacy should immediately be separately organized," the original Shenzhou Medicine and Pharmacy Association (*Shenzhou yiyao xuehui* 神州醫藥學會)[1] reorganized itself in accordance with the edict as the "Medical Culture Organization (*Yiji de wenhua tuanti* 醫界的文化團體)." However, not long afterwards, the government again instructed that it, "make a trial-run of merging with the Chinese Medicine Association (*Zhongyi xiehui* 中醫協會)," but this aroused a great deal of dissatisfaction among the committee members of the original Shenzhou Medicine and Pharmacy Association. Within the profession, people generally felt that there was no way to "join together a scholarly and a professional organization, their natures are completely unlike." Therefore, in August 1930, by means of

---

1 Historically, medicine and pharmacy were so tightly connected that the term "medicine and pharmacy (*yiyao* 醫藥)" is often best translated simply as "medicine" but here a distinction is being made.

© KONINKLIJKE BRILL NV, LEIDEN, 2020 | DOI:10.1163/9789004420724_022

a resolution of the Fourth Unified Oversight Congress (*Disi jianlian zhixi hui* 第四監聯執席會), it was requested that the government "rescind the order" which had not yet been ratified. Not only this, the Nationalist government once again issued an edict in October of the same year, stating, "According to reports from this districts ten sections, the three organizations—Shenzhou Medicine and Pharmacy Association, the Chinese Medicine Association (*Zhongyi xuehui* 中醫學會), and the United Association of Chinese Medicine and Pharmacy (*Zhonghua yiyao lianhehui* 中華醫藥聯合會)—use outlandish names and are formed improperly. We therefore earnestly command that they merge and reorganize. Please take action accordingly" ("Abstract of the Proceedings of the Shenzhou National Medicine Association—Record of the Members' Conference on Reorganization [*Shenzhou guoyi xuehui huiwu zhaiyao—gaizu huiyuan dahui jilu* 神州國醫學會會務摘要—改組會員大會紀錄]," volume 1, issue 1). Under such a situation, the Shenzhou National Medicine Association was forced to halt all work. Subsequently, through the ceaseless struggles of the Chinese medical community and like-minded people, and with the vocal support of the Association's members, yet another petition jointly presented by "Shenzhou National Medicine Association" and the "Unified Association of Chinese Medicine and Pharmacy" finally succeeded in obtaining the Nationalist government's agreement that the associations need merely reorganize and not merge together. In August 1931, "Shenzhou Medicine and Pharmacy Association" convened a reorganization conference and formally changed its name to "Shenzhou National Medicine Association" (afterwards, "the Association"). This journal also began publication in the first month of that year.

Cheng Diren was from Fujian. He was a famous physician of Shanghai and active in the struggles between Chinese and Western medicine. He was secretary for the Shenzhou Medicine and Pharmacy Association and the Shenzhou National Medicine Association. From 1931 to 1937, he was director of the Association's committee on scholarship and editing. At the same time, he was also director of the official documents division of the general affairs group. On March 17th, 1929, during the National Chinese Medicine Resistance Movement, he participated in the March 17th Shanghai National Medical Organization Representatives Conference and became a managing member of the conference.

Wu Quji, whose dates are unclear, was a modern physician. His works include the book *Xuetang's Medical Discussions* (*Xuetang yiyu* 雪堂醫語). His *Quji's Medical Discussions* (*Quji yihua* 去疾醫話) was serialized in *Shenzhou National Medical Journal* and mostly recorded fantastic stories and unusual occurrences. He explained, "in my spare time from medical practice, I broadly read the various masters and the hundred schools from the pre-Han period, picking out the strange, novel, and heartening among them, and writing them down. It was merely a diversion for myself, but then I had a sudden realization. Therefore, I make bold to speak forth here" ("Editor's Note [*Bianzhe yan* 編者言]," volume 1, issue 6). According to Mr. Shen Zhonggui's 沈仲圭 recollection, in the last years of the Republic, due to the bleak situation of clinical work, Wu Quji became depressed and died (Shen Zhonggui, "How I Learned Chinese Medicine [*Wo shi zenyang xuexi zhongyi de* 我是怎樣學校怎樣的]," in *The Path of Famous Senior Chinese Medicine Physicians* [*Ming laozhongyi zhi lu* 名老中醫之路], China Press of Traditional Chinese Medicine, 2010).

22. National Medicine Bulletin (Guoyi gongbao 國醫公報)

On October 10th, 1932 (the twenty-first year of the Republican period), the *National Medicine Bulletin* was founded in Nanjing. It was edited and published by the secretariat of the Central National Medicine Institute (*Zhongyang guoyi guan* 中央國醫館). This was the official publication of the National Medicine Institute. In December 1936, the last issue was published. Altogether four volumes and thirty-eight issues were published. The first, second, and third volumes each contained twelve issues. Only two issues of the fourth volume were published. Volume 2, Issue 6, and volume 3, issue 4, were special issues. The *National Medicine Bulletin* was intended as a monthly periodical, but the third, fourth, and fifth issues of the first volume were published every other month. For the year of 1934 only two issue were published, labeled volume 2, issues 1 and 2.

The Central National Medicine Institute was formally established on March 17th, 1931, in Nanjing. Chen Lifu 陳立夫 was the chairman of the board of directors, which was composed of ten people, including Peng Yangguang 彭養光, Lu Yuanlei 陸淵雷, and Xie Liheng 謝利恆. Jiao Yitang 焦易堂 was the president of the Institute. Chen Yu 陳郁 and Shi Jinmo 施今墨 were the Institute's vice-presidents. The Central National Medicine Institute was modern Chinese medicine's first national education institution. The Institute President, Jiao Yitang (1880–1950), was named Ximeng 希孟 but went by the courtesy name Yitang. He was from Wugong county, Shaanxi. He was a graduate of the law division of Beijing's Chinese Public School (*Zhongguo gongxue* 中國公學). As a youth he followed Mr. Sun Yat-sen (Sun Zhongshan 孫中山), joined the United League of China (*Tongmeng hui* 同盟會), and participated in the 1911 Revolution. After the Nanjing government was established, he was a member of the legislative council. Jiao Yitang was originally found of and familiar with traditional Chinese medicine and fought a lengthy battle against the erroneous actions of Wang Jingwei 汪精衛 and others who wanted to "abolish Chinese medicine and prohibit the use of the National medicinals." He made a great contribution to the protection and development of Chinese medicine. The *National Medicine Bulletin* operated under the guiding principle of "making Chinese medicine scientific." It energetically upheld Chinese medicine's legal status, systematized and organized Chinese medicine, and developed Chinese medical pedagogy. The "Introduction" to the inaugural issue, observed, "It is appropriate that we do our utmost to catch up [to Western medicine],

© KONINKLIJKE BRILL NV, LEIDEN, 2020 | DOI:10.1163/9789004420724_023

energetically improve, promote the ancient learning, absorb the new learning, assemble the knowledge and ability of specialists, return to the fundamental system of Chinese medicine, learn from each other's successes and failures, and see together and hear together so that we may flourish ever more day by day. The possibility of bringing actual benefit to society depends on it. This is this institute's mission in publishing the *National Medicine Bulletin*. I hope that every member of the national medical community can exert themselves for it."

23. Contemporary Medicine Monthly (Xiandai yiyao yuekan) 現代醫藥月刊 (Contemporary Medicine [Xiandai yiyao 現代醫藥])

In May 1933 (the twenty-second year of the Republican period), *Contemporary Medicine Monthly* was founded in Fuqing county, Fujian. Yu Shenchu 俞慎初 was the first editor-in-chief. Wen Jingxiu 溫敬修, Li Jianyi 李健頤, and Chen Yingqi 陳應期 were special contributors. It was published by the Contemporary Medicine Society (*Xiandai yiyaoxue she* 現代醫藥學社). Starting with volume 2, issue 1, the journal's name on the cover changed to *Contemporary Medicine*. From volume 1, issue 1, to volume 3, issue 2, this journal was a monthly publication; however, in volume 1, issues 6 and 7, 8 and 9, and 10 and 11, were published as combined bimonthly issues. Starting with volume 3, issue 3, this journal began to publish one issue per week. Each issue was only one page and was carried in the *Fuqing People's Bulletin* (*Fuqing minbao* 福清民報) on page four. Presently available material for this journal stops at volume 4, number 11 (March 16th, 1937).

The editor-in-chief, Yu Shenchu (1915–2002) was originally named Jin 謹. His pen name was Jingxiu 靜修. He was a Chinese medical physician from Fuqing county, Fujian. When he was young, Yu Shenchu studied medicine with Qin Bowei 秦伯未. In 1933 he graduated from the Shanghai College of Chinese Medicine (*Shanghai zhongyi xueyuan* 上海中醫學院). After the founding of the New China, Yu Shenchu became a professor at the Fujian College of Chinese Medicine (*Fujian zhongyi xueyuan* 福建中醫學院). He was chosen as a national-level expert on Chinese medicine, one of the One Hundred Famous Chinese Medical Clinicians of the Century, and one of the Teachers for Guiding the Work of Carrying on the Learning and Experience of the Senior Chinese Medical Physicians of the Entire Country.

In the 1930s, Yu Shenchu was interested in the eastward flow of Western knowledge and found the intellectual atmosphere of Chinese medicine itself to be sluggish. Moreover, the development of Chinese medicine was restricted by the government. Influenced by the many famous physicians who were systematizing learning, founding medical associations, or publishing medical journals, he formed the Contemporary Medicine Society and edited and published *Contemporary Medicine Monthly*.

Like other Chinese medical scholarly organizations, the Contemporary Medicine Society was directed against the academic situation state of affairs that many people were infatuated with Western studies and attacked Chinese medicine and the social reality that the development of Chinese medicine was suffering from government restrictions. "Our idea of sociability is to exert ourselves to aid in this critical situation." "We embrace the mission of research and advocacy, promoting the national essence and advancing new knowledge." "We are engaged in organizing our own medicine." "... in order that it can accomplish its purpose of aiding the world and saving lives" ("The Contemporary Medicine Society's Publishing Manifesto [*Xiandai yiyao xueshe fakan xuanyan* 現代醫藥學社發刊宣言]," volume 1, issue 1).

The journal's title was usually written in the hand of a famous physician from the Chinese medical community. The entire first volume as well as volume 2, issues 4 through 6, and volume 3 were penned by Jiao Yitang 交易堂, president of the Central National Medicine Institute. In the blank space at the top of the covers of volume 2, issues 7 through 12, were written by Chen Lifu 陳立夫. Volume 2, issue 4, through volume 3, issue 2, the motto "Examine the Past, Grasp the Present, Build the Future" was written. On the left edge of the covers of volume 2, issues 4 through 6, "Critiquing the Merits and Drawbacks of Chinese and Western Studies from the Point of View of Truth" as a statement of the editor's pragmatic and truth-seeking attitude.

24. Acumoxa Magazine (Zhenjiu zazhi 針灸雜誌)

On October 10th, 1933 (the twenty-second year of the Republican period), *Acumoxa Magazine* began publishing in Wuxi, Jiangsu. Cheng Dan'an 承淡安 was the editor-in-chief, and the Chinese Acumoxa Research Association (*Zhongguo zhenjiu xue yanjiuhui* 中國針灸學研究會) published and distributed it. It originally was a bimonthly magazine publishing six issues per year, but from volume 3, issue 1, onward, it became a monthly magazine. It ceased publication with the outbreak of the War of Resistance against Japan.[1] Altogether, it published thirty-five issues. In 1951, it resumed publication and released six issues. Its name was then changed to *Acumoxa Medicine* (*Zhenjiu yixue* 針灸醫學). Altogether, it published fifteen issues.

Cheng Dan'an (1899–1957) was also called Dan'an 澹盦. He was from Jiangyin, Jiangsu, and was a famous acupuncturist. He began studying medicine with his father at the age of seventeen. From assisting with patients to trying his hand at examining them on his own, he studied for three years, after which he had grasped Chinese medical theory and clinical knowledge. In 1919, he studied internal medicine with his fellow Wuxi-native, Qu Jianzhuang 瞿簡莊. By means of this intensive study he advanced rapidly. He built a sturdy foundation for his later advanced studies. In 1920, he joined the Shanghai Chinese-Western Medicine Correspondence School (*Shanghai Zhong-Xi yi hanshou xuexiao* 上海中西醫函授學校) as a student and got a handle on some Western medical diagnostic techniques.

In the winter of 1921, Cheng Dan'an returned home and practiced medicine with his father. In the course of clinical practice he realized that many difficult and puzzling illnesses could be treated with acumoxa and cured. He developed a great interest in the study of acumoxa and assiduously studied the *Numinous Pivot* (*Lingshu* 靈樞), the *Classic of Supporting Life with Acumoxa* (*Zhenjiu zisheng jing* 針灸資生經), and the *Great Compendium of Acumoxa* (*Zhenjiu dacheng* 針灸大成). He specialized in acupuncture techniques and modern knowledge of physiology and anatomy. In 1925, he began practicing medicine on his own. He ran a clinic independently in the Pishi and Wangting, Suzhou, using acumoxa as his primary means of treating illness.

In 1930, Cheng Dan'an founded the Chinese Acumoxa Research Society in Wangting and became its president. This was the first acumoxa educational structure teaching by correspondence in the history of Chinese medical education. In 1932, the Chinese Acumoxa Research Society's headquarters moved

---

1 World War II.

© KONINKLIJKE BRILL NV, LEIDEN, 2020 | DOI:10.1163/9789004420724_025

to 56 Hangtou Shang, Nanmen Wai, Wuxi. After strengthening the teaching materials and revising the method of recruiting students, the number of students from inside the country and overseas increased daily. While running the school, Cheng Dan'an wrote *A Record of the Cheng Lineage's Experience with Acumoxa* (*Chengmen zhenjiu shiyan lu* 承門針灸實驗錄) and gave it to students for free. In October 1933, Cheng Dan'an founded *Acumoxa Magazine*. This was the first magazine devoted to acumoxa in Chinese history. The contributors to this magazine were primarily members of the society from many places as well as practitioners or students of acumoxa. Starting in 1934, the Chinese Acumoxa Research Society set up clinical practicums. Students who came to study with the society were required to spend five months in clinical study. The clinical practicum program was held twice every year. This society integrated the study of acumoxa theory and clinical practice. They also set up a column in *Acumoxa Magazine* to publicize the students' accomplishments.

In the autumn of 1934, Cheng Dan'an moved to Japan to study and research for eight months. While in Japan, Cheng Dan'an ran about everywhere collecting Japanese acupuncture teaching and research materials as well as acumoxa instruments. He looked through acumoxa texts which were seldom seen in China but circulating in Japan. Among them he found the *Illustrated Study of the Channels and Points according to the Bronze Man* (*Tongren jingxue tukao* 銅人經穴圖考) and Hua Boren's 滑伯仁 *Exposition on the Fourteen Channels* (*Shisi jing fahui* 十四經發揮), which had long been lost in our country. Through his efforts, these precious texts which had been lost were found again.

In 1935, after Cheng Dan'an returned from Japan, he decided to establish a school using the Chinese Acumoxa Research Association as the foundation and established the Chinese Acumoxa Institute (*Zhongguo zhenjiu jiangxisuo* 中國針灸講習所). He also published his complete edited and punctuated version of the old text of *Exposition on the Fourteen Channels* in volume 3, issue 6, of *Acumoxa Magazine*. The headquarters of the Chinese Acumoxa Research Society then moved once more, this time to Yanqiaoxia, Xishuiguan, Wuxi. In February, 1937, the Chinese Acumoxa Institute changed its name to the Chinese Acumoxa Medical School (*Zhongguo zhenjiu yixue zhuanmen xuexiao* 中國針灸醫學專門學校). With their unceasing development, more than three thousand students completed a course of study at the Chinese Acumoxa Research Society or the Institute/Medical School. In 1937, with the outbreak of the War of Resistance against Japan, this journal temporarily ceased publication.

After the establishment of the New China, the government placed great emphasis on acumoxa. In 1951, the Chinese Acumoxa Research Society resumed operation on Siqian Street in Suzhou. *Acumoxa Magazine* was also able to resume publication. In 1954, the Jiangsu provincial government invited Cheng Dan'an to become president of the Provincial Chinese Medicine Advanced Studies School (*Zhongyi jinxiu xuexiao* 中醫進修學校) (the predecessor of Nanjing University of Chinese Medicine [*Nanjing zhongyiyao daxue* 南京中醫藥大學]). Shortly thereafter, he was selected to be a member of the first department of education of the Chinese Academy of Sciences (*Zhongguo kexue yuan* 中國科學院). Cheng Dan'an poured all of his enthusiasm and effort into acumoxa theory, clinical practice, teaching, and research as well as the training of skilled Chinese medical doctors. He trained a large cohort of elite doctors to make Chinese acumoxa the world's leader in acumoxa. Over the course of several decades he personally taught several thousand people and taught more than ten thousand people by correspondence. His students were spread across the entire country and also the countries of Southeast Asia. Not a few of them have become expert professors and famous scholars both here and abroad.

25. Guanghua Medical Magazine (Guanghua yiyao zazhi 光華醫藥雜誌)

On November 15th, 1933 (the twenty-second year of the Republican period), *Guanghua Medical Magazine* was founded in Shanghai. It was edited and published by the Guanghua Medical Magazine Society (*Guanghua yiyao zazhi she* 光華醫藥雜誌社). The society's headquarters was located at #9 Dailongli, West Beishan Road, Shanghai. The journal was printed in high quality at a 16mo size. The journal title on the cover was written by Chen Lifu 陳立夫. Each issue was approximately one hundred pages long. In July 1937, it ceased publication. Altogether, it published forty-five issues.

Ding Zhongying 丁仲英 was the editor-in-chief of this journal. Beginning with volume 1, issue 9, Xie Liheng 謝利恆 became the manager of the "Reader's Association Medical Guidance Section (*Duzhe hui yixue zhidao bu* 讀者會醫學指導部)." Later on, Shen Zongwu 沈宗吳 and others held the post of editor. The directors of the society were ten distinguished personages and members of the Chinese medical community, including Chen Guofu 陳果夫, Chen Lifu, Jiao Yitang 焦易堂, Qin Bowei 秦伯未, and Kong Bohua 孔伯華. Starting with volume 1, issue 10, Tang Jifu 唐吉父 became the society's president. The editor-in-chief and contributors to the magazine were mostly famous practitioners of Chinese medicine in Shanghai at the time, and this journal had profound influence on the Chinese medical community.

The editor-in-chief of this journal, Ding Zhongying (1886–1978), used the courtesy name Yuanyan 元彥. He was the son of the famous modern physician Ding Ganren 丁甘仁 and had authored *A Treatise on Health* (*Kangjian lun* 康健論)—which was rather influential—together with Chen Cunren 陳存仁. In 1911, when the Shanghai Chinese Medicine Association (*Shanghai zhongyi xuehui* 上海中醫學會) was established, he was selected as chairman of the board of directors. He directed the Shanghai Chinese Medicine School (*Shanghai zhongyi zhuanmen xuexiao* 上海中醫專門學校), the Shanghai Chinese Medicine Association (*Shanghai zhongyi xuehui* 上海中醫學會), the Shanghai National Medicine College (*Shanghai guoyi xueyuan* 上海國醫學院), and the Shanghai Chinese Medicine College (*Shanghai zhongyi xueyuan* 上海中醫學院). He became a member of the board of directors of the Central National Medicine Institute (*Zhongyang guoyi guan* 中央國醫館), president of the Shanghai branch of the National Medicine Institute, and a member of the board of directors of the Unified National Association of Medical Organizations (*Quanguo yiyao tuanti zonglian hehui* 全國醫藥團體宗聯合會). The president

© KONINKLIJKE BRILL NV, LEIDEN, 2020 | DOI:10.1163/9789004420724_026

of the Guanghua Medical Magazine Society, Tang Jifu (1903–1986) used the courtesy name Julu 桔廬 and the sobriquet Jifu 吉甫. He was from Huzhou, Zhejiang. In 1919, he studied with the famous Huzhou physician Zhu Guyu 朱古愚. In 1924, he went to Shanghai to practice medicine. He was a teacher in both the China Medical College (*Zhongguo yixueyuan* 中國醫學院) and the New China Medical College (*Xin Zhongguo yixue yuan* 新中國醫學院). In 1956, he became a physician at Shanghai Number One Medical College's Hospital of Gynecology and Obstetrics. (*Shanghai diyi yixueyuan fuchanke yiyuan* 上海第一醫學院婦產科醫院). Later he became director of the department of Chinese medicine. Mr. Tang worked in the departments of internal medicine, skin diseases, gynecology, and pediatrics. He was particularly skilled in gynecology. After 1949, he was successively a member of the board of directors of Chinese National Medical Association (*Zhonghua quanguo yixuehui* 中華全國醫學會), a managing director of the Shanghai branch of the Chinese National Chinese Medicine Association (*Zhonghua quanguo zhongyi xuehui* 中華全國中醫學會), and director of the Shanghai Chinese Medicine Association's Gynecology Committee (*Shanghai zhongyi xuehui fuke weiyuanhui* 上海中醫學會婦科委員會).

The mission of *Guanghua Medical Magazine* was "to advance national medicine, develop our native culture, extend well-being to the mass of the people, help bring about the strengthening of the nation, promote national medicinals, relieve the economic distress of the villages, and resist the aggression of Western pharmaceuticals. These are the conditions of prosperous lives for the people" (volume 1, issue 1). The goals of the journal included reflecting trends in Chinese medical practice, promoting communication within the Chinese medical community, forming a scholarly movement within the Chinese medical community, summarizing the clinical experience of physicians, and spreading Chinese medical knowledge. The journal claimed to be "China's only monthly periodical of medical scientization" (volume 1, issue 1).

26. Contemporary Chinese Medicine (Xiandai zhongyi 現代中醫) (Contemporary Chinese Medicine Magazine [Xiandai zhongyi zazhi 現代中醫雜誌])

In January 1934 (the twenty-third year of the Republican period), *Contemporary Chinese Medicine* was founded by Yu Hongren 余鴻仁 and Chen Huimin 陳惠民 in Shanghai. Initially, Yu Hongren was the editor-in-chief and Chen Huimin was the distributor. The society's [*sic*] headquarters was located at #1, Yirenli, Shipi Lane, Ximen, Shanghai. This journal was published monthly on the first of the month. At the beginning of 1937, Yu Hongren insisted on stepping down from his editorial duties because he was too busy with clinical work. After consultation, Chen Huimin invited his teacher, Ding Jiwan 丁濟萬 to take up the post of society president and himself became editor-in-chief. The journal also changed its name to *Contemporary Chinese Medicine Magazine*. It resumed publication on May 15th. After publishing three issues, the journal ceased publication due to the outbreak of the War of Resistance against Japan. Altogether, it published thirty-nine issues. The fifth through the twelfth issues, in the twenty-fifth year of the Republican period (1936), were paired combined issues. Therefore, this journal altogether published thirty-five physical volumes.

Yu Hongren (1915–1970) was from Changshu, Jiangsu, and was a member of the Menghe medical current (*Menghe yipai* 孟河醫派). He was the grandson of the famous late Qing physician Yu Tinghong 余聽鴻 (Jinghe 景和) and the second son of Yu Jihong 余繼鴻 (Zhenyuan 振元, Weijing 渭經). In 1932, he graduated from Shanghai Chinese Medicine College (*Shanghai zhongyi xueyuan* 上海中醫學院), because he was a student of Ding Jiwan of Menghe, he practiced medicine privately in Shanghai under the name "Menghe Yu Hongren." His older brother Yu Hongsun 余鴻孫 (1906–1956) was the elder son of Yu Tinghong, a student of Ding Ganren 丁甘仁, and a famous physician in Shanghai. While he was pursuing his studies, Mr. Yu began to develop thoughts about innovation in Chinese medicine and collected relevant materials. Not long after graduating, he founded *Contemporary Chinese Medicine* with his schoolmate Chen Huimin. Furthermore, since his family had a strong background in medicine, he had extensive contact and communication with like-minded physicians of the previous generation, such as Qin Bowei 秦伯未 and Chen Cunren 陳存仁, who made it easy for him to found a journal.

© KONINKLIJKE BRILL NV, LEIDEN, 2020 | DOI:10.1163/9789004420724_027

27. Tieqiao's Medical Monthly (Tieqiao yixue yuekan 鐵樵醫學月刊)

In January of 1934 (the twenty-third year of the Republican period), *Tieqiao's Medical Monthly* was founded in Shanghai. It was published under the name of the Tieqiao Correspondence Education Medical Firm (*Tieqiao hanshou yixue shiwusuo* 鐵橋函授醫學事務所) and was edited by Yun Tieqiao's 惲鐵橋 favorite student Zhang Juying 章巨膺. In December 1935, it ceased publication. Although this journal was named a "monthly," over the course of two years it published altogether twenty issues, or ten issues per year.

Yun Tieqiao (1878–1935) was named Shujue 樹珏 and used the sobriquets Lengfeng 冷風, Jiaomu 焦木, and Huangshan 黃山. He was from Menghe, Wujin, Jiangsu. As a child he was orphaned and poor. His father died when he was five. When he was eleven, his mother passed away. A fellow clansman took him in and raised him. At the age of thirteen, he entered a private family school and at sixteen passed the county-level imperial examinations. In 1903 he entered Shanghai Nanyang Public School (*Shanghai Nanyang gongxue* 上海南洋公學) and intensively studied foreign languages and literature. In 1906, after graduating, he worked as a teacher in Changsha, Hunan, and Shanghai. In 1911, he accepted the invitation of the Commercial Press's (*Shangwu yinshuguan* 商務印書館) Mr. Zhang Jusheng 張菊生 to become a translator and editor for the Commercial Press. The following year, he edited *Fiction Monthly* (*Xiaoshuo yuebao* 小說月報), becoming celebrated in the literary world for his translation of foreign stories. He then began to put all of his effort into the study of Chinese medicine, because both his eldest son and his second son one after the other died young from disease. In 1920, he resigned from his editorial work at *Fiction Monthly* and formally hung up his shingle as a practicing doctor specializing in pediatrics. In 1925, he founded the "China Correspondence-Education Society (*Zhongguo tonghan jiaoshou xueshe* 中國通函教授學社)"—which would later become familiar as "Tieqiao's Chinese Medicine Correspondence School (*Tieqiao hanshou zhongyi xuexiao* 鐵橋函授中醫學校)"—with the great scholar of traditional Chinese culture, Zhang Taiyan 章太炎, and his student Zhang Polang 張破浪.

In 1932, Yun Tieqiao began to feel run-down due to overwork. At Zhang Taiyan's invitation, Mr. Yun went to Mr. Zhang's residence in Suzhou to rest and recuperate. When the condition of his health had improved a bit, he returned to Shanghai and continued practicing medicine and running his school.

© KONINKLIJKE BRILL NV, LEIDEN, 2020 | DOI:10.1163/9789004420724_028

Because he overexerted himself, the accumulated fatigue produced an illness, and Mr. Yun's last years were spent paralyzed and bedridden. Even though he was in such a condition, he continued to author books by dictation and never became slack. Finally, since his illness steadily deteriorated, he passed away in Shanghai on July 16th, 1935.

Mr. Yun placed great emphasis on integrating theory and practice. He stressed the importance of absorbing new knowledge on top of a foundation of the learning and experience inherited from previous generations so that one could supplement, improve, and develop Chinese medicine. He felt that if we want Chinese medicine to advance and evolve, we must "elucidate ancient ideas," "incorporate new knowledge," learn from other's strong points to supplement our weaknesses, and "absorb Western medicine's strong points and blend with it so as to reinvigorate Chinese medicine." He believed that both Chinese and Western medicine had their strong points. Chinese medicine values seeing a person in the context of the whole of nature and accords with the changes and transformations produced by the four seasons and yin and yang. In terms of physiology, Western medicine values anatomy, and in terms of pathology emphasizes localized pathological changes. One should be well versed in both types of medicine and take the best from each. At the same time, he stressed that "you absolutely cannot make Chinese medicine assimilate to Western medicine. You can only take Western medicine's principles to supplement Chinese medicine. You can draw strength from elsewhere, but you must not lose yourself in the process" (*Deliberations on Medicine* [*Yixue pingyi* 醫學評議] in *The Medicine Box Medical Book Series* [*Yi'an yixue congshu* 醫盒醫學叢書]).

Mr. Yun lived at precisely the time when Chinese and Western culture were beginning to interact. Most of those practicing medicine neglected the study of theory and emphasized collecting formulae for specific conditions. It reached the point that it was as if the Chinese medical classic, the *Yellow Emperor's Inner Classic* (*Huangdi neijing* 黃帝內經), had been placed on a high shelf and was seldom the subject of inquiry. Mr. Yun started from the point of view of upholding the scientific nature of the system of Chinese medical theory. By analyzing the essence of the theory of the *Inner Classic*, he was able to explicate in a rather complete fashion those aspects fundamental Chinese medical theory—yin and yang, the five phases, the six *qi*, etc.—which people found difficult to understand. From the point of view of methodology, Mr. Yun revealed the essential character of the system of Chinese medical theory. He clearly and explicitly explained the primitive dialectical awareness of Chinese medical thought.

Among Mr. Yun's closer personal students, the more influential—such as Zhang Juying, Xu Hengzhi 徐衡之, Gu Yushi 顧雨時, He Gongdu 何公度, Lu Yuanlei 陸淵雷, and Zhuang Shijun 莊時俊—all became the backbone of the future Chinese medical community.

The editor-in-chief, Zhang Juying (1899–1972), who was also named Shoudong 壽棟, was from Jiangyin, Jiangsu. At a young age he apprenticed with a teacher to study medicine. In 1919, he became an editor in the Shanghai Commercial Press's translation department. In his free time he broadly read medical books and studied Chinese medicine on his own. In the fourteenth year of the Republican period, he became Yun Tieqiao's student and experienced great progress. After three years his studies were complete and he set up a clinic in Zhabei. In a short while he became well-known. Mr. Zhang studied the *Treatise on Cold Damage* (*Shanghan lun* 傷寒論) very deeply and made a contribution to our understanding of it. In regard to the cold damage and damp-heat categories of illnesses, he developed a new point of view in regards to "theory, method, formulas, and herbs."[1] Clinically, he used medicinals flexibly, and was the first to develop the method of treating measles with a mist-like spray of Chinese medicinals.

---

1   I.e., all aspects of the clinical process.

28. Suzhou National Medicine Magazine (Suzhou guoyi zazhi 蘇州國醫雜誌)

In March 1934 (the twenty-third year of the Republican period), *Suzhou National Medicine Magazine* was founded in Suzhou. It was published and distributed by the Suzhou National Medicine Society (*Suzhou guoyi xueshe* 蘇州國醫學社). Tang Shenfang 唐慎坊 was the society's president, and Wang Shengan 王慎幹 was the general director. Hu Xiaowu 胡蕭梧, Ye Juquan 葉橘泉, Wang Nanshan 王南山, Zhou Baiqiang 周白強, Chen Danhua 陳丹華, and Zhang Youliang 張又良 were special contributors. It was printed by Suzhou Wenxin Printing House (*Suzhou wenxin yinshuguan* 蘇州文新印書館). This journal was printed seasonally in a 16mo printing format. It primarily published transcriptions of lectures, papers, and medical cases of famous physicians of Chinese and western medicine as well as papers written by students of the society. It also published some longer Chinese medical texts and class lecture notes in serial form as well as translations of Japanese texts on Chinese medicine. In December 1936, this journal ceased publication. Altogether it published twelve issues.

Suzhou National Medicine Society's predecessor was the Suzhou Women's Medicine Society (*Suzhou nuke yishe* 蘇州女科醫社) founded by Wang Shengan. In the autumn of 1933, the Women's Medicine Society expanded and changed its name to Suzhou National Medicine Society. In the winter of 1934, it became the Suzhou National Medicine School (*Suzhou guoyi xuexiao* 蘇州國醫學校). Later it again changed its name, becoming the Suzhou National Medicine Training School (*Suzhou guoyi zhuanke xuexiao* 蘇州國醫專科學校) and also founded the Suzhou National Medicine Research Institute (*Suzhou guoyi yanjiuyuan* 蘇州國醫研究院). Tang Shenfang was the president of the school and Wang Shengan was the vice-president and general director. Zhang Taiyan 章太炎 was invited to become the honorary president of the school and president of the research institute. Zhang Taiyan gave periodic lectures to the teacher and students.

Wang Shengan (1900–1984) was from Shaoxing, Zhejiang. He was a contemporary Chinese medical physician and educator. As a youth, he graduated from Zhejiang's Number Five Teacher's School. In 1916, he became a student of the famous Shanghai physicians Ding Ganren 丁甘仁, Cao Yingfu 曹穎甫, and Huang Tiren 黃體仁. He was one of the early students of Ding Ganren's Shanghai Chinese Medicine School (*Shanghai zhongyi zhuanmen xuexiao* 上海中醫專門學校). In 1924, he moved to Suzhou and opened a private clinic,

© KONINKLIJKE BRILL NV, LEIDEN, 2020 | DOI:10.1163/9789004420724_029

becoming well-known for his skill in women's medicine throughout Jiangsu, Zhejiang, and Shanghai. In 1926, he founded the Suzhou Women's Medicine Society. Over the course of seven years four classes of students graduated, or approximately seven hundred people from all of the provinces of the country as well as the Malay archipelago. In 1933, the "Suzhou Women's Medicine Society" changed its name to the "Suzhou National Medicine Society." In 1954, after the establishment of the New China, Wang Shengan accepted a position as director of the Jiangsu Provincial Chinese Medicine Improvement School (*Jiangsu sheng zhongyi jinxiu xuexiao* 江蘇省中醫進修學校) (the predecessor of Nanjing Chinese Medicine University [*Nanjing zhongyiyao daxue* 南京中醫藥大學]) as well as clinic director for the Chinese Medicine School's clinic. He participated in the compilation and proofreading of *An Outline of Chinese Medicine* (*Zhongyixue gailun* 中醫學概論) and was the chief proofreader of *Concise Chinese Medical Gynecology* (*Jianming zhongyi fukexue* 簡明中醫婦科學). At the end of the 1950s and the beginning of the 1960s, these two books had a tremendous impact on Chinese medical education. In 1957, he moved to Beijing and took a teaching position at Beijing College of Chinese Medicine (*Beijing zhongyi xueyuan* 北京中醫學院). He participated in the draft discussions and proofreading of second higher learning edition of *Chinese Medical Gynecology* (*Zhongyi fukexue* 中醫婦科學) as well as Beijing College of Chinese Medicine's *Teaching Materials on Gynecology* (*Fukexue jiangyi* 婦科學講義) and *Theories of the Various Schools of Chinese Medicine* (*Zhongyi gejia xueshuo* 中醫各家學說). He made a great contribution to the writing and editing of the unified textbooks for the entire country's Chinese medicine schools.

29. Correct Words on National Medicine (Guoyi zhengyan 國醫正言)

In June 1934 (the twenty-third year of the Republican period), *Correct Words on National Medicine* was founded in Tianjin. It was Tianjin's earliest Chinese medicine periodical. Chen Zengyuan 陳曾源 was the editor-in-chief, and Zhou Wei 周偉, Sun Mingshan 孫鳴山, Shen Xiaoqing 沈肖卿, Zhao Duansheng 趙端升, Zhao Hansong 趙寒松, Qi Zhixue 齊志學, and Zhang Lanting 張蘭亭 were successively editors. It was published by the Tianjin Municipal National Medicine Research Association (*Tianjin shi guoyi yanjiuhui* 天津市國醫研究會) and printed by Tianjin Benefit the World Newspaper Office (*Tianjin yishi baoguan* 天津益世報館). This journal was a monthly periodical. Starting with June 1934, it was published on the first of every month. In 1937, after the "July 7th" incident,[1] it was forced to cease publication. Altogether it published thirty-eight issues. It also published one collection, the *Omnibus Volume* (*Huiding ce* 彙訂冊), gathering together the content of the first through the twelfth issues. In the *Omnibus Volume*, the first section includes the Hunan physician, Zeng Juesou's 曾覺叟, "Forward to the Collected Articles of Tianjin's *Correct Words on National Medicine*."

The general purpose of this journal was to promote national medicine and national medicinals as well as save lives. The opening article of the inaugural issue was Chen Zengyuan's "Manifesto (*Xuanyan* 宣言)," in which he states, "Nowadays, human feeling is too hollow. In this generation whose desire for personal profit is so great, Chinese medicine is troubled of its own within and Western medicine is invading from without. Therefore, the true Way of Qibo and the Yellow Emperor[2] is gradually perishing. We must have a firm and indomitable will and protect it with all our strength. Only then will it be able to continue saving lives for all time. Although my medical knowledge is meager, I am willing, for the sake of those who uphold the teachings of Qibo and the Yellow Emperor, to see to it that other currents of medicine are unable to invade and destroy it. For that reason, I am gathering together like-minded physicians who are honest and upright to form a periodical that will be a

---

1 The beginning of the Japanese invasion of China and the War of Resistance against Japan (World War II).
2 Qibo and the Yellow Emperor are the principal interlocutors in the *Yellow Emperor's Inner Classic (Huangdi neijing* 黃帝內經), which is traditionally seen as the founding document of Chinese medicine; hence, Chinese medicine as a whole.

© KONINKLIJKE BRILL NV, LEIDEN, 2020 | DOI:10.1163/9789004420724_030

mechanism for the protection of the teaching of Qibo and the Yellow Emperor. I have therefore named it '*Correct Words on National Medicine*.'" From this we can see the resolution of Chen Zengyuan's vow to be a protector of the teachings of Qibo and Huangdi. He engaged in vigorous activity to make this journal a mechanism for protecting the teachings and exerted himself to the utmost in disseminating the correct Way of Chinese medicine in order to benefit the people and promote the national essence. This is truly the origin and meaning of this journal's title, *Correct Words on National Medicine*.

The editor-in-chief, Chen Zengyuan (1873–1939) used the courtesy name Yidong 譯東 and the religious sobriquet "Reaches to the Original (*Dayuanzi* 達元子)." He was from Tianjin and was a modern Chinese medical physician and educator. At the age of eighteen, he passed the exams to become a student at the Imperial College in the capital. He changed his studies from Confucian scholarship to medicine because members of his family had died from the incorrect treatment of incompetent doctors. The main books he authored include, *Examining National Medicine's Cold Damage Theory* (*Guoyi shanghan keyi* 國醫傷寒課義), *Teaching Materials on Medicine* (*Fangmai jiangyi* 方脈講義), *Teaching Materials on Warm Disease* (*Wenbing jiangyi* 溫病講義), *The Medical Classics on the Principles of Life and Health Preservation* (*Yijing shengli weisheng xue* 醫經生理衛生學), *Annotations and Explanation of Cold Damage* (*Shanghan zhujie* 傷寒注解), *Elucidating the Classics on Women's Diseases* (*Nübing chanjing* 女病闡經), and *Heart Classic of the Throat* (*Yanhou xinjing* 咽喉心經). Mr. Chen was not only skilled at medical technique, he also energetically threw himself into Chinese medical education. Moreover, he raced up and down the country raising a ruckus to secure the legal status of Chinese medicine, carrying out an indomitable struggle. He felt that cultivating talented individuals was the most important aspect of promoting Chinese medicine. Therefore, in addition to practicing medicine, he established a private family school and taught the medical classics to some of the students. At that time it was truly pioneering work. A few practicing physicians were also interested enough to come and attend his lectures. In 1927, Mr. Chen petitioned the Zhili provincial education department for permission to open the Tianjin City Private Chinese Medicine Training Institute (*Tianjin shi sili zhongyi chuanxisuo* 天津市私立中醫傳習所). This was Tianjin's earliest private Chinese medicine school as well as one of the earliest private Chinese medicine schools in the entire country. Mr. Chen personally became president of the training institute as well as undertaking teaching duties. He also personally edited the teaching material, *Examining National Medicine's Cold Damage Theory*, which was published serially in *Correct Words on Chinese Medicine*. The instruction at the training institute was strict and the academic atmosphere upright. It's reputation in the Tianjin Chinese medical community was extremely good. Its graduates all went on to become the backbone of the medical community of the time, like Li Runtian 李潤田, Sun Shaoshan 孫少山, Chai Pengnian 柴彭年, Xing Chunlin 邢春林, Bao Shusheng 鮑樹生, Bao Wenbing 鮑文柄, Song Xiangyuan 宋向元, Song Yuming 宋宇鳴, Wu Yusun 吳玉蓀, Zhang Gongzhuo 張共琢, Zhang Juying 張聚英, Zhao Wenlu 趙文祿, Wang Chenguang 王晨光, and Ji Liangchen 紀良臣. Afterwards, all of them were famous in Tianjin. In 1939, Mr. Chen developed a severe illness, but continued to teach from his sickbed until the last moments of his life. Afterwards, his second son, Chen Shichun 陳士純, continued running the school. In 1941, when Chen Shichun passed away, the school ceased operation.

In the Republican period, the Chinese medical community encountered many difficulties. It was full of ups and downs in every way possible. In order to save Chinese medicine in its time of troubles, many famous Chinese medical physicians rose to the fight and raced about raising an uproar. Mr. Chen was one of these. In February 1929, at the first meeting of the central health committee convened by the department of government's health department in Nanjing, Yu Yan 余岩 and others submitted "A Proposal for Abolishing Old Medicine in order to Clear away Obstacles to Medicine and Health (*Feizhi jiuyi yi saochu yishi weisheng zhang'ai an* 廢止舊醫以掃除醫事衛生之障礙案)" and it was approved. This is the "Proposal to Abolish Chinese Medicine" infamous in modern Chinese medical history. As news of it spread, it aroused the wrath of the entire country's Chinese medical community, and they rose up to fight against it. Mr. Chen was the first member of the Tianjin Chinese medical community to vigorously respond to it. Mr. Chen brought together the famous physicians of the city and the province under the banner of the Tianjin Chinese Medicine Trade Association (*Tianjin zhongyi gonghui* 天津中醫公會). On March 17th, the "Unified National Association of Medical Associations (*Quanguo yiyao tuanti lianhehui* 全國醫藥團體聯合會)" was established in Shanghai and separately approached the Third National General Congress (*Disanci quanguo daibiao dahui* 第三次全國代表大會), the Executive Institute (*Xingzheng yuan* 行政院), the Legislative Institute (*Lifa yuan* 立法院), the Health Department, and the Education Department. They also individually presented petitions and demonstrated to make known their determination to save Chinese medicine from extinction. In March 1931, the Central National Medicine Institute (*Zhongyang guoyi guan* 中央國醫館) was established with Jiao Yitang 焦易堂 as its president. He vigorously defended the rights of Chinese medicine. In July of the same year, Mr. Jiao presided over the forty-third meeting of the legal institution committee (*fazhi weiyuanhui* 法制委員會) of the Legislative Institute and drafted the "Regulations for National Medicine (*Guoyi tiaoli* 國醫條例)." Afterwards its name was changed to "Regulations for Chinese Medicine (*Zhongyi tiaoli* 中醫條例)." For a wide variety of reasons, these regulations were laid to one side and never granted a hearing. In an excess of righteous indignation, Mr. Jiao resigned his positions as a legislative committee member, chair of the legal institutions committee, and president of the National Medicine Institute. On hearing this news, Mr. Chen felt that Mr. Jiao was the hard-to-obtain core strength of the Chinese medical community. Having thought it over from the big picture, he used his position as chair of the Tianjin Chinese Medical Trade Association to petition the Central Legislative Institute, exhorting the government to persuade Mr. Jiao to remain in his former positions. "in order to inspire the able and virtuous, protect national medicine, and guard the affairs of our race." In January 1936, "Regulations for Chinese Medicine" was finally promulgated and put into effect. It was a safeguard for the development of Chinese medicine.

30. Chinese Medicine's New Life (Zhongyi xin shengming 中醫新生命)

In August 1934 (the twenty-third year of the Republican period), *Chinese Medicine's New Life* was founded in Shanghai. It was managed by Lu Yuanlei Medical House (*Lu Yuanlei yishi* 陸淵雷醫室). Lu Yuanlei was the director and publisher. Xie Songmu 謝誦穆 was the editor. This journal was a monthly periodical in the 32mo printing format. It was published at the end of every month. After the thirtieth issue, Xie Songmu resigned as editor because of his father's passing. The periodical was obliged to delay its publication, struggling to publish one issue every two months. It only sustained itself for two issues and then announced that it was ceasing publication. Over the course of two-and-a-half years, it published altogether thirty-one issues.

Lu Yuanlei Medical House opened a correspondence education program. Participants increased day by day. In order to make it easy for classmates to examine one another's questions and answers to the homework, *Record of the Transmission and Learning of the New Chinese Medicine* (*Xin zhongyi chuanxi lu* 新中醫傳習錄) was printed. However, on reading it, Mr. Lu felt that it having gone through "the process sending out an edited school publication, it would be a waste of effort if it were only read by accepted students." Therefore, he changed the name to *Chinese Medicine's New Life* with the purpose of "using Chinese medicinal substances to treat illness and scientific principles to research its methods and principles" ("Notice Inviting Contributions to this Journal," number 1). He broadly sought contributions and sold the journal both within the country and without. Because the first issue was already printed, it was inconvenient to make many changes. Therefore, the header of the pages still read "*Record of the Transmission and Learning of the New Chinese Medicine.*"

The editor, Xie Songmu, used an English saying in the "Introduction": "The inexhaustible treasures of the world were buried for those that will seek them." He thought that regardless of whether one is old or young, if one strives greatly and moves forward with an indomitable will, this can be called "youth." The treasures of Chinese medicine require the youth to exert their intelligence in seeking them. Only then will there be progress; only then will there be hope of rejuvenation. Therefore, he chose the name "*Chinese Medicine's New Life.*"

Lu Yuanlei (1894–1955) was named Pengnian 彭年 and was from Chuansha district, Shanghai. As a youth he was clever and bright and devoted to his studies. Later on, he studied with the great master of textual studies (*puxue*

© KONINKLIJKE BRILL NV, LEIDEN, 2020 | DOI:10.1163/9789004420724_031

樸學), Yao Mengxun 姚孟醺, becoming drunk on the study of the classics and the lesser learning (*xiaoxue* 小學). He also studied with Zhang Taiyan 章太炎 and the famous physician Yun Tieqiao 惲鐵樵. In 1928, he taught at the Shanghai Chinese Medical School (*Shanghai zhongyi zhuanmen xuexiao* 上海中醫專門學校) and the Shanghai China Medical School (*Shanghai Zhongguo yixueyuan* 上海中國醫學院), researching the theories of famous Chinese medical physicians. In 1928, together with Xu Hengzhi and Zhang Cigong, he founded the Shanghai National Medicine College (*Shanghai guoyi xueyuan* 上海國醫學院) and became its dean of studies. He took "elucidate ancient ideas and incorporate new knowledge" as his motto in running the school. He took the lead in incorporating physics, chemistry, and anatomy in the curriculum, and also wrote the teaching materials *A Modern Explanation of the Treatise on Cold Damage* (*Shanghan lun jinshi* 傷寒論今釋) and *A Modern Explanation of Essentials of the Golden Coffer* (*Jingui yaolue jinshi* 金匱要略今釋), using a contemporary medical point of view to explicate the Chinese medical classics. Starting in 1932, he opened a medical practice in Shanghai, using Western medical techniques of diagnosis but prescribing classical formulae as treatment. He was particularly skilled at treating cold damage and other epidemic febrile diseases as well as chronic hepatitis and tumors. The same year, at the request of students from all directions, he opened a correspondence school under the name "Lu Yuanlei Medical House." Before long, he had students from everywhere within the country and also Southeast Asia. In the teaching materials, which he prepared himself, he blended and linked the Chinese and the Western and were meticulously presented. Jiang Chunhua 姜春華 and Yue Meizhong 岳美中 both received his instruction. In 1934, he founded the magazine, *Chinese Medicine's New Life*, in order to call for the scientization of Chinese medicine. The articles directly refuted Yu Yunxiu's 余云岫 defamations of Chinese medicine. His words were fierce, responding point for point to the "Abolishing Chinese Medicine Current (*Zhongyi feizhi pai*)." People acclaimed him as "both erudite and thunderous." It was also said, "The Western medical community has Mr. Yu Yunxiu. The Chinese medical community has Mr. Lu Yuanlei. They are both able to enter the tiger's den in search of tiger cubs.[1] You can truly say they are well-matched" ("A Letter from Jin Zhenyu 金正愚 of the Railway Ministry," issue 3). After the founding of the People's Republic, Lu Yuanlei at various times was vice-chair of the Shanghai Municipal Medical Science Research Committee (*Shanghai shi yikexue yanjiu weiyuanhui* 上海市醫科學研究委員會), chair of the Shanghai Municipal Chinese Medicine Association (*Shanghai shi zhongyi xuehui* 上海市中醫學會),

---

1   I.e., they are willing to brave great risks in order to gain great rewards.

Chinese medicine consultant to the Shanghai Municipal Department of Public Health (*Shanghai shi weishengju* 上海市衛生局), and director of the Shanghai Chinese Medicine Clinic (*Shanghai zhongyi menzhensuo* 上海中醫門診所). He was also selected as a representative to the National People's Congress. In 1954, he oversaw the editing of Chinese medical teaching materials. In 1955, he became the chair of the Shanghai College of Chinese Medicine Hospital Preparation Committee (*Shanghai zhongyi xueyuan choubei weiyuanhui* 上海中醫學院籌備委員會). The following year he died due to illness. Mr. Lu writings are voluminous. Apart from the two "*Modern Explanation*" books mentioned above, he also wrote *Mr. Lu's Collected Writings* (*Lu shi jilun* 陸氏集論), *An Explanation of the Chinese Medical Physiology Terminology* (*Zhongyi shengli shuyu jie* 中醫生理術語解), *An Explanation of Chinese Medical Pathology Terminology* (*Zhongyi bingli shuyu jie* 中醫病理術語解), *Essentials of Epidemic Disease* (*Liuxing bing xuzhi* 流行病須知), *An Outline of the Treatise on Cold Damage* (*Shanghan lun gaiyao* 傷寒論概要), and *Essential Guidance on Tongue Diagnosis* (*Shezhen yaozhi* 舌診要旨).

Xie Songmu (1912–1973) was also named Zhongmo 仲墨. He was from Xiaoshan, Zhejiang. He graduated from Shanghai National Medicine College and studied with Lu Yuanlei, researching Zhang Zhongjing's 張仲景 *Treatise on Cold Damage and Miscellaneous Disease* (*Shanghan zabing lun* 傷寒雜病論). He participated in the editing of and also studied from the two "*Modern Explanation*" books. Later on, he became a teacher at the Shanghai Chinese Medicine Correspondence School (*Shanghai zhongyi hanshou xuexiao* 上海中醫函授學校) and edited the magazine, *Chinese Medicine's New Life.* He also assisted in resolving the difficult questions of the correspondence students. In 1936, because Qiu Jisheng 裘吉生 was growing old and weak, Xie Songmu accepted an invitation to become editor-in-chief of the *Triple-Three Medical Journal* and also oversaw the preparation of the printing of the *Triple-Three Medical Book* (*San-san yishu* 三三醫書). In 1937, he returned to his hometown and practiced medicine there. Toward the end of 1955, he, along with the famous contemporary physician Shen Zhonggui 沈仲圭, accepted the invitation of the Ministry of Health to move to Beijing and take a position at the Chinese Academy of Chinese Medicine (*Zhongguo zhongyi yanjiuyuan* 中國中醫研究院). His publications include *A Critical Evaluation of Warm Disease* (*Wenbing lunheng* 溫病論衡), *The Essential Meaning of Warm Disease* (*Wenbing yaoyi* 溫病要義), *An Examination of Spurious Texts* (*Weishucong kao* 偽書叢考), and *An Examination of Spurious Chinese Texts* (*Zhonghua weishu kao* 中華偽書考).

31. Beiping Medical Monthly (Beiping yiyao yuekan 北平醫藥月刊)

In January of 1935 (the twenty-fourth year of the Republican period), *Beiping Medical Monthly* was founded in Beiping. It was edited and published by the Beiping Medical Monthly Society (*Beiping yiyao yuekan she* 北平醫藥月刊社). The president of the society was Yang Jieru 楊洁如. The title of the journal was written in the calligraphy of the president of the Central National Medicine Institute (*Zhongyang guoyi guan* 中央國醫館), Jiao Yitang 焦易堂. This was a monthly journal. In total, it published three issues. The contributions to the magazine were mostly written by Beiping Medical Monthly Society members. There were more than thirty members of the society including Fang Xingwei 方行維, Fang Boping 方伯屏, Kong Bohua 孔伯華, Kong Zhonghua 孔仲華, Wang Shengwu 王省吾, Wang Shutian 王澍田, Zuo Jiyun 左季雲, An Ganqing 安幹卿, Li Gechi 李革痴, Wang Dachun 王逢春, Xu Yichen 徐逸塵, Chen Yishi 陳以時, Sun Xianglin 孫祥麟, Zhang Zichang 張子暢, Zhang Juren 張菊人, Zhang Jianfeng 張劍逢, Cao Yangzhou 曹養舟, Fu Fengshan 傅佩珊, Yang Shucheng 楊叔澄, Yang Jieru 楊如, Yang Xiaoping 楊筱坪, Ye Juanqing 葉狷卿, Guan Wenru 管文如, Zhao Shuping 趙樹屏, Deng Hepeng 鄧鶴朋, Liu Yanong 劉亞農, Liu Hanchen 劉翰臣, Han Yiqi 韓一齊, and Xiao Longyou 蕭龍友.

Yang Jieru (1881–1940) was named Dejiu 德九. He was from Huaiyin county in Jiangsu province. He was a famous modern Chinese medicine physician. He was born in a family of hereditary Chinese medical doctors and was accepted as a student by the famous local physician Yang Shishou 楊世壽. Yang Jiru enjoyed teaching others. As a youth, he assisted the imperial governor of Shandong, Yang Shixiang 楊士驤, establish a Chinese medical school. In 1910, after he moved to Beijing, he became head physician of the Outer City Official Physician's Office (*Waichengguan yiyuan* 外城官醫院). The medical goals of the Official Physician's Office were limited. In order to be able to treat more commoners, Yang Jiru resigned as head official physician and opened Beijing's first private Chinese medical hospital, "Yang Jielu's Chinese Medicine Hospital (*Yang Jielu zhongyiyuan* 楊洁盧中醫院)," and saved the lives of many patients of common origins, earning the respect of the people. The Beiping Medical Monthly Society was established in Yang Jilu Chinese Medicine Hospital.

Yang Jiru, in the introduction to this journal, introduced the conditions that gave rise to the this journal: "I regretted that our medicine was gradually declining without hope of renewed vigor. Some students lacked teachers;

© KONINKLIJKE BRILL NV, LEIDEN, 2020 | DOI:10.1163/9789004420724_032

others lacked systematicity. It was dissipating day by day. At this rate, it would inevitably be ruined and afterwards cease to exist." Therefore, publishing this journal could not be delayed. "It so happened that the Beiping National Medicine College's (*Beiping Zhongguo yixueyuan* 北平國醫學院) summer vacation had passed, and we were holding the opening ceremonies for the sixth semester. Famous scholars wee assembled in a single hall." They were all extremely anxious about the development of Chinese medicine and were willing to make concerted efforts together to promote the development it. "It was decided to get together over a meal twice each month to facilitate discussion and carefully distinguish the nature of the situation in hopes of arriving at the highest principal and most essential words as a contribution to society and to assist with the inadequacy of scholarship." Apart from this, in the dedication for this journal, Cao Longyou analyzed the necessity of founding this journal. He thought that Chinese medicine was vast and profound, there were transmissions through families and through teachers; therefore, it was difficult to create a system. Furthermore, there was an esoteric section of Chinese medicine. Although it had effective medicines and remarkable formulae, it was not transmitted to outsiders. This had led to the loss of many secret formulae and proven formulae. Therefore, "in light of this situation, my colleagues and I have established a research association and are also publishing a monthly journal. We hope to elucidate the ancient knowledge, write it down in books, and provide it collectively. When among modern patients, there are puzzling and difficult cases, we will explain the nature of the illness and its treatment method. If there is a cure, it must be clinically corroborated. If a cure has not been found, we can diagnose together to find an effective remedy. By uniting like-minded people throughout the country in this way, we can learn from one another, exchange information, ensure that secret formulae that are no longer being transmitted are made known through this journal, and effective treatment methods are circulated by means of it. When the transmission and learning of knowledge are already old, then the virtuosos appear. We must corroborate our origins and gradually form them into a system so that our learning can progress and our efforts have a basis. Once sincerity lifts up its head, the many virtues are already prepared." The Medical Monthly Society brought together many renowned people of integrity. Most of them were famous Beiping physicians. Some of them taught at the Beiping National Medicine College. Others were simultaneously involved in in other journal societies. The influence of their scholarship was rather strong. This journal was founded to carry forward Chinese medical culture and encourage Chinese medicine's continued development and application of its positive purpose.

32. Chinese-Western Medicine (Zhongxi yiyao 中西醫藥)

In August 1935 (the twenty-fourth year of the Republican period), *Chinese-Western Medicine* was founded in Shanghai. It was edited by the Shanghai Chinese-Western Medical Research Society. Chu Minyi 褚民誼, Wu Liande 伍連德, and Zhu Hengbi 朱恆璧 wrote the journal title in their calligraphy. This was a monthly journal published in the 16mo printing format. In August 1937, it ceased publication for the first time. In October 1946, it resumed publication. In December 1947, it ceased publication a second time. Altogether it published thirty-eight issues. The Education Ministry of the Communist Party cabled orders that the entire country's medical and health offices should subscribe to it. This journal's standing board of directors was Ding Fubao 丁副保, Song Daren 宋大仁, and Guo Qiyuan 郭琦元. The departments of scholarship, general affairs, and publishing that were established beneath them managed the specific concerns of the journal. The person responsible for each department was, respectively, Zhu Hengbi, Shen Jingfan 沈警凡, and Song Daren. beneath each department a number of sections were also established.

Song Daren and others began forming the Chinese-Western Medical Research Society in 1932. After three years of preparation, on January 26th, 1935, it was formally established. The guiding principles of this society were: to gather together China's skilled medical professionals and research Chinese and Western medicine in order to bring about the improvement of Chinese medical scholarship; to scientific methods to research medicine, make truth our only goal, and reject the private views of the various factions; to vigorously inculcate a knowledge of health and medicine among the masses, in order to bring about the rejuvenation of the Chinese people's inherent spirit health ("This Society's Constitution [*Benshe zhangcheng* 本社章程]," volume 1, issue 1). The domain of the society's activities included the following areas: to research Chinese medical history; to introduce new knowledge of practical relevance to health and medicine; to test, cultivate, and identify nationally produced medicinals; to network with other scholarly organizations and cooperate in researching medicinals; to investigate statistically the medical situation; to gather together old medical books and historical resources; to discuss the problem of medical progress; to inculcate everyday knowledge of health among the masses; to stand firm in legal disputes over medicine and safeguard the profession; to publish a monthly periodical and medical texts; to prepare

© KONINKLIJKE BRILL NV, LEIDEN, 2020 | DOI:10.1163/9789004420724_033

for the establishment of the Shanghai Circulating Medical Library (*Shanghai liutong yiyao tushuguan* 上海流通醫藥圖書館) ("This Society's Cause and the Rights of Entering the Society [*Benshe shiye yu rushe quanli* 本社事業與入社權利]," volume 1, issue 1). Apart from this, in order to understand the trend of each country's medical development, society members from outside China were invited to make on-the-spot inspections and submit reports so that medical advancements in every country would arrive appear before the faces of the readers in a timely fashion ("A Record of this Society's Establishment and its Current Situation [*Benshe chengli jingguo ji ji jinkuang* 本社成立經過記及近況]," volume 1, issue 1). Since, in the society of the times, the debate between Chinese and Western medicine was growing more intense by the day, this society broadly included medical specialists from the entire country, embraced the idea that scholarship has no borders, took the search for truth as its culture, used scientific methods to research medicine, hoped to put an end to disputes, and standardized theories.

33. Cultured Medicine Semimonthly (Wenyi banyuekan 文醫半月刊)

On December 1st, 1935 (the twenty-fourth year of the Republican period), *Cultured Medicine Semimonthly* was founded in Beiping. Shi Jinmo 施今墨 was the director. Shi Jinmo, Chen Bocheng 陳伯誠, and Yang Yiya 楊益亞 were the chief editors. They also invited Yang Shucheng 楊叔澄, Wang Xiaoxian 王孝先, and Wang Zongzhe 王宗喆 to be advisers and Zhang Cunying 張存英, Guo Manzhi 郭曼之, Li Heyi 李和義—all personages from the Chinese medical community—to be special contributors. It was published and distributed by the North China National Medicine College Cultured Medicine Semimonthly Society (*Huabei guoyi xueyuan wenyi banyuekan she* 華北國醫學院文醫半月刊社). This journal was published semimonthly on the first and sixteenth of every month. Each issue was approximately sixteen pages in length and printed in a 16mo printing format. After July 1st 1937, it ceased publication. Altogether it published four volumes and thirty-seven issues.

The cover of this journal changed several times. For the first three issues of the first volume, one-third of the cover was occupied by the journal title, volume and issue numbers, and the publication date. The left and right margins displayed the price and the society's address. The remaining two-thirds contained "This Issue's Table of Contents" (on the first issue this differed, containing the "Introduction [*Fakanci* 發刊詞]"). It was simple and easy to use at a glance. For volume 1, issues 4 through 7, several small changes were made to this basic cover. First, above the title was printed "Mr. Shi Jinmo, Director," as an indication of the journal's authoritative character. Second, the title was written in Shi Jinmo's own calligraphy. Third, for the convenience of readers purchasing it, the locations of the distributors were listed below the table of contents. For volume 1, issues 8 through 12, and volume 2, issues 1 through 5, the typesetting cover changed from top-to-bottom to format to left-to-right. The title and table of contents occupied half of the cover and the location of the distributors was listed below them. Beginning with volume 2, issue 6, the title was written in the calligraphy of Jiao Yitang 焦易堂. Starting with volume 3, issue 3, the cover displayed the journal's English title. As for setting up columns, for the first thirteen issues, few columns were established and moreover, they were not particularly fixed. For the remaining twenty-four issues, the number of established columns increased. Only volume 3, issues 7 and 8, were published as a combined issue.

© KONINKLIJKE BRILL NV, LEIDEN, 2020 | DOI:10.1163/9789004420724_034

Shi Jinmo (1881–1969) was originally named Yudian 毓點 and hometown was Xiaoshan, Zhejiang. He was a Chinese medical clinician and educator and one of the "Four Great Physicians of Beiping (*Beiping sida mingyi* 北平四大名醫)." He worked tirelessly his whole life for the Chinese medical profession, insisting on the Chinese medical practice of determining treatment by pattern differentiation (*bianzheng lunzhi* 辨證論治) and advocating the integration of Chinese and Western medicine. His clinical efficacy was remarkable. In 1931, the Central National Medicine Institute (*Zhongyang guoyi guan* 中央國醫館) was established, and he became its vice-president. He founded the Beiping National Medicine College (*Beiping guoyi xueyuan* 北平國醫學院) with the famous physicians Xiao Longyou 蕭龍友, Kong Bohua 孔伯華 and became its vice-president. In 1932, he founded the North China National Medicine College (*Huabei guoyi xueyuan* 華北國醫學院) with Wei Jiangong 魏建宏, Liu Zhaozhen 劉肇甄, and Chen Gongsu 陳公素 and became its president. In 1941, he became the chair of the board of directors of the Shanghai Fuxing Chinese Medicine Training School. He trained many talented Chinese medical physicians, successfully treated many puzzling and difficult syndromes, formulated many new medicines, and offered up seven hundred proven formulae. He made a surpassing contribution to the Chinese medical profession and has a remarkable reputation inside and outside of the country. His clinical experience can be seen in *Shi Jinmo's Medical Cases Selected by Mr. Zhu* (*Zhu xuan Shi Jinmo yi'an* 祝選施今墨醫案) and *A Collection of Shi Jinmo's Clinical Experiences* (*Shi Jinmo linchuang jingyan ji* 施今墨臨床經驗集).

The other two editors, Chen Bocheng and Yang Yiya, both graduated from North China National Medicine College. Afterwards, they became professors there and spent many years teaching and researching Chinese medicine. Their work on cold damage and formula studies was particularly profound. They also played an important role in publishing and publicizing of periodicals.

34. National Medical Literature (Guoyi wenxian 國醫文獻)

In the spring of 1936 (the twenty-fifth year of the Republican period), *National Medical Literature* was founded in Shanghai. It was edited by this journal's editorial committee and published and distributed by the Shanghai City National Medicine Trade Association (*Shanghai shi guoyi gonghui* 上海市國醫公會) and the Shanghai Chinese Medicine College (*Shanghai Zhongguo yixueyuan* 上海中國醫學院). This was a seasonal journal. On the basis of what can now be seen, it only published two issues, spring and summer. This journal was simultaneously the association journal of the Shanghai City National Medicine Trade Association and the college journal of the Shanghai Chinese Medicine College. According to "Report on the Business of the National Medicine Trade Association (*Guoyi gonghui huiwu baogao* 國醫公會會務報告)" in volume 1, issue 2, in the first meeting of the joint committee of provisional office-holders at the seventh plenary members conference that took place on January 18th, 1936, there was a proposal "the general assembly communicates its request to found a research night school and revive the association's periodical." The results of the discussion of this proposal at the time were, "It is decided: management of the night school will be handed over to the Chinese Medicine College. The association's journal has at present already been revived. We can see that at the latest, the magazine, *Chinese Medical Literature*, was founded by January 1936.

The editorial committee of *Chinese Medical Literature* was formed from the members of the National Medicine Trade Association, the board of directors of the Chinese Medicine College, as well as all of its professors. Its publishing organization—Shanghai Chinese Medicine College—was founded in 1927 by the Shanghai National Medicine Trade Association. Zhang Taiyan 章太炎 was the first president. The famous Chinese medicine physicians Qin Bowei 秦伯未, Jiang Wenfang 蔣文芳, Bao Shisheng 包識生 supported its activities. In 1932, after the "January 28th Incident,"[1] the school's debts piled up. Zhu Hegao 朱鶴皋 accepted management of it. At that time it was "stipulated that within five years, we will resume the responsibilities taken on individually by the gentleman Zhu. The trade association will not be able to interfere in management during this period. When the time is complete, accounts will be settled and the management of the school will return to the trade association. Within that period, any profits and losses will, without exception, have no bearing

---

1 The date of an early Japanese attack on the Zhabei district of Shanghai.

© KONINKLIJKE BRILL NV, LEIDEN, 2020 | DOI:10.1163/9789004420724_035

on the trade association," "we have chosen a person to handle administration and entrusted him with complete authority" ("Report on the Conditions of the Affairs of the Trade Association [*Guoyi gonghui huiwuqing bao* 國醫公會會務情報]," volume 1, issue 1). In October 1935, before the expiration of the specified period, Zhu Hegao resigned from all of his relevant duties. The National Medicine Trade Association "in view of the fact that the Chinese Medicine College has in fact already become the highest educational institution of national medicine" ("Report on the Conditions of the Affairs of the National Medicine Trade Association," volume 1, issue 1), resumed management of the college and appointed Xue Wenyuan 薛文元 as its president. Guo Bailiang 郭柏良 and others were vice-presidents. Xia Yingtang 夏應堂 was the chair of the board of directors. Xie Liheng 謝利恆, Chen Cunren 陳存仁, Qin Bowei, and Bao Shisheng were directors. Ye Jingqiu 葉勁秋, Xu Xiaopu 徐小圃, and Xu Banlong 許半龍 all taught courses there. According to text of the relevant previously cited articles in volume 1, issue 1, of this journal, the school had more than three hundred students at the time. In December of the year Zhu Hegao resigned, he again made preparations for another Chinese medicine school, named the "New Chinese Medical College (*Xin Zhongguo yixueyuan* 新中國醫學院)." In actuality, students and teachers often moved among the several Chinese medicine schools in Shanghai at the time.

35. Mainstay of National Medicine Monthly (Guoyi dizhu yuekan 國醫砥柱月刊)

In January 1937 (the twenty-sixth year of the Republican period), *Mainstay of National Medicine Monthly* was founded in Beiping. Yang Yiya 楊醫亞 was the president of the cooperative as well as editor and publisher. It was published by the Mainstay of National Medicine Monthly Society (*Guoyi dizhu yuekan she* 國醫砥柱月刊社). It was a monthly publication in the 16mo printing format. A full year of twelve issues was counted as one volume. Each issues content averaged around sixty pages. This journal ceased publication in September 1948. Altogether it published six volumes and seventy-two issues.

Yang Yiya (1914-?) was originally named Yang Yiya 楊益亞. He was from Wenxian, Henan. His family was poverty-stricken. In 1934 he successfully entered the famous modern physician, Mr. Shi Jinmo's 施今墨, "Beiping's North China National Medicine College (*Huabei guoyi xueyuan* 華北國醫學院)." In his second year there, he became a member of Mr. Shi Jinmo's Cultured Medicine Semimonthly Society (*Wenyi banyuekan she* 文醫半月刊社) and practiced the work of editing under the guidance of his advisor. In 1937, he came to feel that the variety of contemporary Chinese medical magazines was too limited and their circulations too small to successfully popularize and improve Chinese medical theory and communicate Chinese medical clinical experience. In this way, the idea of creating a leader among magazines first occurred to him. Therefore, he resolutely founded *Mainstay of National Medicine Monthly*. In 1939, in order to cultivate and train skilled Chinese medical doctors, he founded the "China National Medicine Correspondence Training School (*Zhongguo guoyi zhuanke hanshou xuexiao* 中國國醫專科函授學校)" and the "Chinese Acupuncture Research Institute Correspondence Training Class (*Zhongguo zhenjiu yanjiusuo hanshoubu xuexiban* 中國針灸研究所函授部學習班)" in Beijing, recruiting in total more than two thousand students. Because he had a method for running his schools, their influence in the country was significant. In 1943, he became a professor of cold damage at Beijing North China National Medicine College. In 1949, he became the president of North China National Medicine College. At various times he had also taught at Hebei Chinese Medicine School (*Hebei zhongyi xuexiao* 河北中醫學校) and Tianjin Medicine School (*Tianjin yixuexiao* 天津醫學校). Yang Yiya placed great emphasis on the unearthing and sorting out of proven folk remedies and formulae proven by experience. He organized and published *Prescriptions from the Qing Imperial Medical Office (Qing taiyiyuan peifang* 清

© KONINKLIJKE BRILL NV, LEIDEN, 2020 | DOI:10.1163/9789004420724_036

太醫院配方) and *A Collection of Chinese Medical Proven Formulae* (*Zhongyi yanfang huibian* 中醫驗放彙編). He also gathered together and organized formulae related to measles, acupuncture, arthritis, and gynecology, bringing them together to form *Formulae Worth One Hundred Thousand Gold* (*Shiwan jin fang* 十萬金方). In 1974, he published the two-part book *A Selection of Chinese Medical Proven Formulae* (*Zhongyi yanfang huixuan* 中醫驗放彙選) on internal medicine and skin diseases. Yang Yiya wrote industriously his entire life and made a positive contribution to the promotion of the medical art of Qibo and the Yellow Emperor.[1] In total, he edited or wrote more than forty Chinese medical texts, many of which are still extant. They are admired by the medical world both nationally and internationally.

In his "Introduction to this Journal (*Chuangkanci* 創刊辭)," Yang Yiya points out: "The degradation of our country's medicine has already reached an extreme state ... Were it not that in regard to our national medicine, the people of our nation have proceeded first from a failure to understand, then advanced to scornful neglect, before finally evolving into a desire to destroy it, how could the degeneration have gotten so out of hand." He felt that under the impact of Western medicine, Chinese medicine was increasingly being looked down on by Chinese people. From "neglect" to "a desire to destroy it," they had slipped to the brink of disaster. He faced this perilous situation and determinedly "fought against the tide of disaster," and founded *"Mainstay of National Medicine Monthly."* "It was my purpose embrace a will of unsurpassed steadfastness, a heart that is undaunted by setbacks, and selflessness in order to research in a pure fashion our country's native medicine ... and restore our country's inherent glory, so as to establish a foundation that will endure for ten thousand generations." He unequivocally stated that his purpose in founding this journal was to call forth "the wisdom and effort of the multitude" of like-minded people from the medical community "to forge ahead together"—to make this journal "a firm rock in midstream."[2]

---

1 Qibo and the Yellow Emperor are the principal interlocutors in the *Yellow Emperor's Inner Classic* (*Huangdi neijing* 黃帝內經), which is traditionally seen as the founding document of Chinese medicine; hence, Chinese medicine as a whole.

2 In Chinese, the term "mainstay (*dizhu* 砥柱)" evokes the image of a rocky island that stands in the middle of the Yellow River's rapids. This phrase is a reference to that image.

36. Chinese Medicine (Zhongguo yixue 中國醫學)

On July 1st, 1937 (the twenty-sixth year of the Republican period), *Chinese Medicine* was founded in Shanghai. It was published by the Chinese Medicine Magazine Society (*Zhongguo yixue zazhi she* 中國醫學雜誌社) and printed by the Chinese Medical Press (*Zhongguo yixue shuju* 中國醫學書局). The society's headquarters were located at #30, Alley 830, Beijing Road, Shanghai. The society's president was Tang Jifu 唐吉父. The general manager was Cui Tixian 崔逷先. The directors of the reader's guidance department were Xiao Tui'an 蕭退庵, Xia Libin 夏理彬, and Yin Zhenyi 殷震一. The director of the reader's service department was Qiu Zhizhong 邱治中. The editors were Shi Jiqun 施濟群, Yu Datong 俞大同, Qin Bowei 秦伯未, Fang Gongpu 方公溥, Sheng Xinru 盛心如, and Zhang Huailin 張懷霖. This was a monthly periodical in the 16mo printing format. Unexpectedly, it only published two issues. The outbreak of the "August 13th Incident"[1] came to an abrupt end.

Tang Jifu (1903–1986) used the courtesy name Julu 桔廬 and the sobriquet Jifu 吉甫. He was from Huzhou, Zhejiang. In 1919, he studied with the famous Huzhou physician Zhu Guyu 朱古愚. In 1924, he went to Shanghai to practice medicine. He treated illnesses of internal medicine, skin diseases, gynecology, and pediatrics, but was especially skilled at gynecology. Before the founding of the People's Republic, he was a teacher in both the China Medical College (*Zhongguo yixueyuan* 中國醫學院) and the New China Medical College (*Xin Zhongguo yixue yuan* 新中國醫學院). In 1952, he founded the Shanghai Laozha District Number One Unified Clinical Services Society (*Shanghai Laozha qu diyi lianhe zhenliao fuwushe* 上海老閘區第一聯合診療服務社). In 1956, he became a physician at Shanghai Number One Medical College's Hospital of Gynecology and Obstetrics. (*Shanghai diyi yixueyuan fuchanke yiyuan* 上海第一醫學院婦產科醫院). Later he became director of the department of Chinese medicine. He was also director of the Shanghai Chinese Medicine Association's Gynecology Committee (*Shanghai zhongyi xuehui fuke weiyuanhui* 上海中醫學會婦科委員會) and was also promoted to become a professor.

---

1   The outbreak of war with Japan.

37. Journal of New Chinese Medicine (Xin zhongyi kan 新中醫刊)

On September 1st, 1938 (the twenty-seventh year of the Republican period), the *Journal of New Chinese Medicine* was founded in Shanghai. The famous physician Zhu Xiaonan 朱小南 was the president of the Journal of New Chinese Medicine Society, which published it. It was represented by Jiaojing Mountain Study (*Jiaojing shanfang* 校經山房) (which was located on Sima Road in Shanghai). It was printed in a 32mo printing format and published thirty-four issues in total.

This journal continuously refined itself through a process of exploration and learning. If we take the cover as an example, initially, the cover displayed the table of contents without separating columns from other content. Beginning with issue 5, the table of contents on the cover showed the names of specific columns. After becoming a semimonthly journal following issue 7, the table of contents appeared in the form of "Highlights," and the complete table of contents appeared on the inside of the cover. The cover table of contents took up the function of recommending particular articles. The final pages, inside back cover, and back cover were primarily used to publish advertisements. They were mostly Chinese medical advertisements, such as "Xu Zhongdao's National Medicinal Company (*Xu Zhongdao guoyao hao* 徐重道國藥號)," "Zhang Hengde's National Medicinal Company (*Zhang Hengde guoyao hao* 張恆德國藥號)," "Lei Yunshang's Hall of Fragrant Recitation Medicine Shop (*Lei Yunshang songfen tang yaopu* 雷允上誦芬堂藥鋪)," and "Fragrant Mountain Hall National Medicinal Company (*Xiangshan tang guoyao hao* 香山堂國藥號)." There were also Harmonious Prosperity Tobacco Firm's (*Hexing yan gongsi* 和興烟公司) advertisements for "Red Sister (*Hongmei* 紅妹)" cigarettes, scientific instrument stores, and some advertisements of physician's hours and locations.

The Journal of New Chinese Medicine Society's structure and use of human resources also gradually improved. At first, its human resources consisted of the president Zhu Xiaonan, the editor-in-chief Zhu Mei 朱沫, the general manager Rong Zhiwen 榮質文, the publisher Fu Xuchu 傅旭初, and the accountant Mao Yue 茅玥. In 1939, in order to increase work efficiency, new features of the work were developed. The journal became semimonthly. Because of this, the inside cover of the twelfth issue announced, "The content has been enriched; caution used in choosing sources; stress laid on editing old medical books; modern literature introduced, clinical experience reported; and new

© KONINKLIJKE BRILL NV, LEIDEN, 2020 | DOI:10.1163/9789004420724_038

discoveries about medicinals verified. The layout has also been changed to a new format, the proofreading made particularly strict, and the punctuation improved. The length will double, and we are also considering raising the price. We plan to sell each issue for one *jiao* and a year's subscription for only one *yuan* of the national currency."[1] This announcement made clear the Journal of New Chinese Medicine Society's rigorous and serious attitude toward publishing. At the same time, the staff of the Journal of New Chinese Medicine Society underwent definite changes. The editorial department went from the original five people to ten people. Zhu Xiaonan remained the president as before. Bao Tianbai 包天白 became an honorary editor. Zhu Zhongde 朱中德 and Yu Weinan 余蔚南 became editors. Rong Zhiwen and Luo Yaoxiang 羅耀祥 became managers. Fu Xuchu took charge of publishing. Shen Zhongru 沈仲如 took charge of advertisements. Mao Jitang 茅濟棠 became the accountant, and Xia Mingyang 夏名揚 took charge of distribution (see the colophon of volume 2, issue 1). The editorial office also moved from the original location—#19, Huayuan Road, Wangjiasha, Shanghai—to #31, Alley 809, Aiwenyi Road. The publication office was located at #76, Limei Road, Fazujie, Shanghai. It was also distributed in Shanghai from Five Continent Press (*Wuzhou shuju* 五洲書局), China Book Company (*Zhongguo tushu shuju* 中國圖書公司), Chinese Medicine Press (*Zhongyi shuju* 中醫書局), and Literary Virtue Press (*Wende shuju* 文德書局) and outside of Shanghai by Hong Kong World Press (*Xianggang shijie shuju* 香港世界書局). In 1940, there were changes to the staff of the editorial department. It increased to eighteen people. Zhu Xiaonan remained the president as before. Bao Tianbai remained an honorary editor. Zhu Zhongde and Yu Weinan became editors-in-chief. Wang Hongshou 王宏綬, Mao Zhixiang 茅志祥, Meng Keming 孟克明, and Gu Xiaoqiu 顧小秋 became editors. Fu Xuchu and Shen Fengming 沈鳳鳴 took charge of publishing. Shen Zhongru and Xu Fugang 徐傅剛 took charge of advertisements, and Mao Jitang and Jin Ming 金明 became accountants (see the colophon to volume 2, issue 9).

In December 1940, in order to suit the needs of every like-minded fellow researcher both nationally and internationally, the Journal of New Chinese Medicine Society sought presidents and members for branch societies in many places ("Notice: The Journal of New Chinese Medicine Society is Seeking Presidents and Members for Branch Societies [*Xin zhongyi kan she zhengqiu gedi fenshezhang ji sheyuan qishi* 新中醫刊社徵求各地分社長及社員啟事]," volume 3, issue 5 combined issue). In 1941, the Journal of New Chinese Medicine Society invited Shen Zongwu 沈宗吳, Shen Xiaogu 沈嘯谷, Jin Shaoling 金少陵, Shi Ruxin 施汝新, Shi Jiqun 施濟群, Zhang Cigong 章次公,

---

1   One *jiao* is one-tenth of one *yuan*.

Zhang Juying 章巨膺, Zhu Weiju 祝味菊, Zhang Yi'an 張易安, Zhuang Wenfang 莊文芳, Tong Shaofu 童紹甫, Qian Jinyang 錢金陽, Qian Gongxuan 錢公玄, Huang Baozhong 黃寶忠, Li Chengchu 勵承初, and Ju An 鞠安 to be special contributors. The scope and influence of the journal was continuously increasing. The society's president, Zhu Xiaonan (1901–1974), was the eldest son of the famous physician Zhu Nanshan 朱南山. At the age of twenty he opened a private medical practice in Shanghai. He was skilled at treating internal medicine, skin diseases, gynecology, and pediatrics. In his middle-age, he became famous as a doctor of gynecology.

38. Beijing Medical Monthly (Beijing yiyao yuekan 北京醫藥月刊)

On January 15th, 1939 (the twenty-eighth year of the Republican period), *Beijing Medical Monthly* was founded in Beijing by the National Medicine Professional Branch Association of the capital guidance section of the New People's Congress (*Xinmin hui* 新民會) formed by the Japanese puppet regime. Wang Fengchun 汪逢春 was the chair of the national medicine profession subcommittee and invited Zhao Shuping 趙樹屏 and An Ganqing 安幹青 to become editors-in-chief. Yang Jieru 楊洁如, Zhang Juren 張菊人, Wang Shiqing 王石清, Zhang Jiwu 仉即吾, Duan Menglan 段夢蘭, Wu Xiuchuan 吳秀川, and Zhang Binren 張賓人 were editors. This journal was largely contributed to by members of the branch of the National Medicine Association (*Guoyi fenhui* 國醫分會) to "give expression to the profound and share their strengths and insights." At the end of the journal there was also an introduction to the association. This was a monthly journal, coming out on the fifteenth of every month. On August 15th, 1939, the eight issue was published. The ninth and tenth issues were published as a combined issue in 1930 [*sic*].[1] The specific sections pertaining to each month cannot be distinguished. From the material currently available, this journal appears to have published only ten issues.

Wang Fengchun (1884–1949) was name Chaojia 朝甲 and used the sobriquet Fengchun 鳳椿. He was from Suzhou, Jiangsu. At first, he studied for the examinations. Later, he studied medicine with the famous Suzhou senior physician Ai Buchan 艾步蟾. On reaching maturity, he moved to Beijing and practiced medicine privately for fifty years, becoming one of "the four great physicians of Beijing (*Beijing sida mingyi* 北京四大名醫)." He energetically devoted himself to Chinese medical education throughout his life, particularly emphasizing training talented individuals and promoting on-the-job training. In 1938, since the National Medicine Trade Association (*Guoyi gonghui* 國醫 公會)—of which Zhang Jiwu was the chair of the board of directors—had, owing to financial difficulties, turned its back on the great principle of nationalism and reorganized to form the New People's Congress's National Medicine Professional Branch Association, Wang Fengchun was selected to be the association's president. At the same time, he made preparations were made for the founding of *Beijing Medicine Monthly*. He personally did the editorial work

---

1 This is presumably a typo for "1940."

while also writing for the journal. Mr. Wang was particularly skilled at treating seasonally-caused illnesses and illnesses of the stomach and intestines. He also elucidated many aspects of damp-warmth disease. His most important writings include, *Chinese Medical Pathology* (*Zhongyi binglixue* 中醫病理學) and *Bolu's Medical Cases* (*Bolu yi'an* 泊盧醫案).

39. A New Voice on National Medicinals (Guoyao xinsheng 國藥新聲)

On April 1st, 1939 (the twenty-eighth year of the Republican period), *A New Voice on National Medicinals* was founded in Shanghai. It was funded by the New Asia Medicinal Factory (*Xinya yaochang* 新亞藥廠) and Ding Fubao 丁福保 was invited to become the editor-in-chief. The New Voice on Chinese Medicinals Society (*Guoyao xinsheng she* 國藥新聲社) published and distributed it. The society's headquarters were located at #3, Alley 1093, Xinzha Road, Shanghai. This journal was a monthly periodical, coming out on the first of each month. On January 1st, 1944, the final issue was published. In total, fifty-nine issues were published.

Ding Fubao (1874–1952) used the courtesy name Zhonggu 仲祜 as well as the courtesy name Meixuan 梅軒. He used the sobriquet Chouyinjushi 疇隱居士. He was from Wuxi, Jiangsu. He was a modern book-collector, physician, and scholar of Buddhism. He studied at Jiangyin Nanjing Academy (*Jiangyin Nanjing shuyuan* 江陰南菁書院). His knowledge was deep and broad, and he read extremely extensively. He was an early example of a scholar who understood both Chinese and Western medicine. He studied mathematics with the famous mathematician Hua Hengfang 華蘅芳 and medicine with the famous physicians Zhang Weiqing 張韋青 and Zhao Yuanyi 趙元益. In the first year of the *xuantong* reign period of the Qing dynasty (1909), in the medical exams of the Imperial Inspectorate held in Nanjing, he obtained the "Outstanding Internal Medicine Physician" certificate. The following year he was sent to Japan to investigate its medical facilities. While in Japan, he also studied at Chida Medical School (*Chida igaku gakkō* 千田醫學學校). When the time came to return to China, Ding Fubao purchased a large number of medical texts. After returning to Shanghai, he opened the Shanghai Medicine Press (*Shanghai yixue shuju* 上海醫學書局) and edited and published more than 160 medical texts from within the country and overseas. The texts he edited included *A Brief Catalogue of Historical Medical Texts* (*Lidai yixue shumu tiyao* 歷代醫學數目提要) and *The Medical Section of the General Record of the Four Divisions* (*Sibu zonglu yibian* 四部總錄醫藥編), with the aim of disseminating the knowledge of Chinese and Western medicine. In the second year of the *xuantong* reign period, he founded the Chinese-Western Medicine Research Association (*Zhong-Xi yixue yanjiuhui* 中西醫學研究會) to advocate for "scientization of Chinese medicine" and promote medical research. He also

© KONINKLIJKE BRILL NV, LEIDEN, 2020 | DOI:10.1163/9789004420724_040

published the *International Medical Journal*. When Ding Fubao was invited to become the editor-in-chief of the new magazine, *A New Voice on Chinese Medicinals*, he was already sixty-six years old. In the "Introduction (*Fakanci* 發刊詞)," he maintained that for forty years he had been integrating Chinese and Western medicine and emphasizing the need to scientize Chinese medicine. He also asserted his deep belief that forty years later the time had come for an integrated Chinese and Western medicine.

40. National Medicine Guide (Guoyi daobao 國醫導報)

In July 1939 (the twenty-eighth year of the Republican period), *National Medicine Guide* was founded in Shanghai. This was a bimonthly magazine run by Shanghai Xinyi Medicinal Factory (*Shanghai xinyi yaochang* 上海信誼藥廠). Zhu Renkang 朱仁康 was the editor-in-chief. It was printed by the Shanghai Chinese Regular Script New-Record Printing House (*Shanghai hanwen zhengkai xinji yinshuguan* 上海漢文正楷新記印書館). On the cover, "National Medicine Guide" was written in the hand of Mr. Ding Jiwan 丁濟萬, and "Choosing the Essence, Selecting the Flowers" was printed in color in seal script. In December, 1941, with the outbreak of the Pacific War, the Japanese occupied and ceased the common concessions, and this journal was forced to cease publication. Altogether, it published three volumes and fifteen issues.

Regarding the purpose of this journal, in the inaugural issue's "Introduction" Zhu Renkang enumerated Chinese medicine's dilatory progress over the last several thousand years: 1) leadership, 2) the limitations of making a living, 3) the lineage point of view, and 4) a complete lack of open collaboration and sharing. He stated that the measures which needed to be put into effect without delay were "putting into order the corpus of Chinese medical texts," "developing our inherent special qualities," "extracting and purifying active components of national medicinals," and "merging of our collective clinical experience." He also made these three items the primary goal of this journal. The following year, in volume 3, issue 1, Mr. Zhu also stressed in his "Forward (*Juantou yu* 卷頭語)": "From today forward, the principles of this journal will remain based on its previous professional guidance. Place no store in unfounded talk; seek only sound scholarship. Do not chase after the profound; seek only the practical. In finding sources, emphasize research articles on the linking up of Chinese and Western medicine. This journal will keep repeating this over and over."

The major contributors to the first issue of this journal were Song Daren 宋大仁, Yan Zhiqing 嚴志清, Qian Jinyang 錢金陽, Xu Boyuan 徐伯元, Yu Ruoping 余若屏, and Lu Qingjie 陸清潔. Afterwards, the journal matured day by day and its reputation increased. Among the ranks of its authors, well-known individuals also increased, including Lu Yuanlei 陸淵雷, Shen Zhonggui 沈仲圭, Yu Wuyan 余無言, Chen Wujiu 陳無咎, Wu Quji 吳去疾, Jiang Chunhua 姜春華, He Gongdu 何公度, Ye Jingqiu 葉勁秋, Bao Juxiang 包句香, Cheng Diren 程迪仁, Qiu Peiran 裘沛然, Zhang Juying 章巨鷹, and Yang Shouren 楊守仁.

© KONINKLIJKE BRILL NV, LEIDEN, 2020 | DOI:10.1163/9789004420724_041

Zhu Renkang (19087–2000) used the courtesy name Xingjian 行健 and the self-chosen sobriquet "Medical Recluse of Liang Creek." He was from Wujin, Jiangsu. He was born in an ordinary city family. Because his family's circumstances were straitened, after studying for one year in junior high, he had to drop out. At the age of seventeen, he began to study medicine with his elder brother. He also studied with the famous skin disease specialist Mr. Zhang Zhikang 章治康. At the age of twenty his studies were completed and he independently opened a clinic in the outskirts of Suzhou. In the early 1930s, he moved to Shanghai, simultaneously running a private clinic and continuing his studies. At that time there was an estrangement between Chinese and Western medicine. Each faction was denouncing the other. They were as incompatible as fire and water. Mr. Zhu felt this was a great pity. He thought that "In regard to Chinese and Western medicine, we cannot emphasize one and neglect the other. It is best if we take in everything, taking the strong points of one to supplement the weak points of the other, combining them to produce an encompassing understanding of both medicines." "Medicine is not divided into Chinese and foreign. In saving a person's life, there is only one Way. Stones from other hills can be used to polish the jade of this one" (preface to *Integrating Chinese and Western Medicine* [*Zhong-Xi yixue huizong—xuyan* 中西醫學匯總·序言]). He used his free time to study Western medicine and systematically studied the lectures Wang Tiyu 汪愓予 wrote for his Chinese-Western medicine correspondence school. At the same time he read broadly in other Western medical books and gathered together study materials. He brought together his many years of clinical realizations to write *Integrating Chinese and Western Medicine* (*Zhong-Xi yixue huizong*), which was published by Shanghai Broad Benefit Press (*Shanghai guangyi shuju* 上海廣益書局) in 1933. Following this, "I practice by taking the Chinese as the center while consulting the Western" became his major theoretical principle in medical practice. Apart from this book, he also wrote *A New Discussion of Skin Diseases* (*Waike xinlun* 外科新論) and *A Modern Explanation of Chinese Medical Terminology* (*Zhongguo yixue zhuanyong mingci jinshi* 中國醫學專用名詞今釋). All of these embodied the Chinese-Western integrated medical point of view that "the Chinese is the essence, the Western is the function." In 1939, Zhu Renkang received the Xinyi Medicinal Factory's invitation to become chief editor for *National Medical Guide*. Before publishing this journal, Xinyi Medicinal Factory had run several periodicals without a fixed publishing schedule. The major contents of *National Medicine Guide* were introductions to this factory's products and their clinical effects. It also published a few academic articles written by specialists or scholars. It was distributed free of charge for doctors from every Chinese and Western medical clinic to read. Zhu Renkang embraced the general principle that "Saving people from illness and suffering is the primary purpose of medicine. There is no inherent difference between new and old. In using medicinals to treat a person's imbalance, where is there a difference between Chinese and Western? It is precisely the case that we can make use of new knowledge to elucidate ancient knowledge" ("Introduction [*Fakanci* 發刊詞]," volume 1, issue 1), so he assumed the heavy responsibility of becoming editor-in-chief. In order to successfully manage this journal, he wore himself out. He managed all of the editorial work almost single-handedly: looking for contributors, correcting submissions, making many friends, and bravely innovating. He made this journal one of the more influential Chinese medicine journals of the day. Mr. Zhu personally wrote many articles. Apart from the introduction, the editor's notes, and the forewords to the volumes, he also wrote many academic and clinical treatises, including "An Explanation of the Six *Qi* and Six Excesses (*Liuqi liuyin quanshi* 六氣六淫詮釋)," *A Modern Explanation of Chinese Medical Terminology*, *A New Discussion of Skin Diseases*, "The Treatment of Anemia through the Liver along with Health Cultivation (*Pinxuezheng gan liaofa ji sheyang* 貧血症肝療法及攝養)."

41. Reviving Chinese Medicine (Fuxing zhongyi 復興中醫)

In January 1940 (the twenty-ninth year of the Republican period), *Reviving Chinese Medicine* was founded in Shanghai. It was founded by the Reviving Chinese Medicine Society. Shi Yiren 時逸人 was the society's president and also the editor. Xu Hongjing 徐鴻經, Yu Shenchu 余慎初, and Shen Zhonggui 沈仲圭 were directors. They also invited Zhu Wenming 朱文明 to be a legal consultant, He Yunhe 何雲鶴 to be a Western medicine consultant, and Li Jusun 李菊蓀 to be an acumoxa consultant. This journal was a monthly publication in the 16mo printing format. One year of six issues was a single volume. It ceased publication in November of the following year. Altogether, it published two volumes and twelve issues.

Shi Yiren (1896–1966) was from Wujin, Jiangsu. He studied Confucian scholarship when young, and became accomplished through self-study. In 1912, he began studying with the famous physician from the same town, Wang Yungong 汪允恭. In 1916, he began practicing medicine privately. In 1926, he founded the "Left Bank National Medicine Institute (*Jiangzuo guoyi jiangxisuo* 江左國醫講習所)"[1] in Shanghai and became a professor at the Shanghai Chinese Medicine School (*Shanghai zhongyi zhuanmen xuexiao* 上海中醫專門學校), a professor at the Chinese Medicine College (*Zhongguo yixueyuan* 中國醫學院), and an editor for *Health Journal* (*Weisheng bao* 衛生報). The following year, he moved to Shanxi to become a member of the standing board of directors for the Shanxi Chinese Medicine Improvement Research Society (*Shanxi zhongyi gaijin yanjiuhui* 山西中醫改進研究會). He edited Shanxi's *Journal of Medicine* (*Yixue zazhi* 醫學雜誌) for almost ten years. After the outbreak of the War of Resistance against Japan,[2] he traveled through Wuhan, Chongqing, and Kunming practicing medicine. In the autumn of 1939, he returned to Shanghai where he taught successively at the Chinese Medicine College, the New Chinese Medicine College (*Xin Zhongguo yixue yuan* 新中國醫學院), and the Shanghai Chinese Medicine Training School (*Shanghai zhongyi zhuanke xuexiao* 上海中醫專科學校). Afterwards, he founded the Reviving Chinese Medicine Training School (*Fuxing zhongyi zhuanke xuexiao* 復興中醫專科學校) with Shi Jinmo 施今墨, Zhang Zanchen 張贊臣, and Yu Shenchu. He was also editor-in-chief

---

1 Referring to the area east of the lower reaches of the Yangtze River, roughly modern Jiangsu province.
2 I.e., World War II.

© KONINKLIJKE BRILL NV, LEIDEN, 2020 | DOI:10.1163/9789004420724_042

for the magazine, *Reviving Chinese Medicine*. Shi Jinmo emphasized gaining a thorough grasp of both Chinese and Western medicine. His writings are particularly abundant, including *Mr. Shi's Studies of the Inner Classic* (*Shishi neijing xue* 施氏內經學), *Mr. Shi's Studies of Prescription* (*Shishi chufang xue* 時氏處方學), and *Mr. Shi's Studies of Physiology* (時氏生理學) among more than ten books. Toward the end of his life, he devoted himself to Chinese medical education and publishing, making a powerful and outstanding contribution to the transmission and development of Chinese medicine.

This journal's cover was written in the calligraphy of Chen Wujiu 陳無咎. In the inaugural issue's "The Reviving Chinese Medicine Society's Declaration of Purpose (*Fuxing zhongyi she xuanyan* 復興中醫社宣言)," it states, "The decline of our country's medicine has already reached a severe degree. The calls for its abolition are already loud in the din of this confused world ... So weighty a matter is worthy of our attention." It takes the causes of the attacks on Chinese medicine to be none other than that "its theory is not scientific, its clinical experience has not been gathered together, its medicinals have not been refined, its clinical practice has not been improved," and the Chinese medical community of the time valued profit above all else, seeking only to seize wealth and horde it. They were completely lax. This was the internal cause of Chinese medicine's fall into such a dangerous situation. The article also stated that the "wreckers" who were willing to be marketers for foreign goods and the "hoarders" who saw medicine as a special secret treasure had become two great obstacles on the path to reviving Chinese medicine. The article stated that Shi Yiren, in order to stir up Chinese medicine would strive to "improve the viewpoint on Chinese medicine and Chinese medicinals" and "establish this magazine as a foundation for the revival of Chinese medicine" by organizing and improving Chinese medical scholarship as the prerequisite in the quest for Chinese medicine's revival. This journal's title, *Reviving Chinese Medicine*, was precisely its guiding principle and purpose.

42. Chinese Medicine Monthly (Zhongguo yiyao yuekan 中國醫藥月刊)

In June 1940 (the twenty-ninth year of the Republican period), *Chinese Medicine Monthly* was founded in Beijing by Tong Demao 董德懋 (he was first the editor-in-chief and later the society president). He invited Shi Jinmo 施今墨 to be a medical consultant and Cao Yingfu 曹穎甫, Lu Yuanlei 陸淵雷, Zhang Cigong 章次公, Shi Yiren 時逸人, Tan Cigong 譚次公, Zhu Huaixuan 祝懷萱, and Wang Jiequan 汪洁權—all famous within the national medical community—to be special contributors. Beijing Chinese Medicine Society (*Beijing zhongyi xueshe* 北京中醫學社) published and distributed it. Initially, it was published and distributed on the fifteenth of every month, but starting with volume 1, issue 4, this was changed to the first of every month. A complete year of twelve issues was one volume. Volume 1, issues 8 and 9, volume 2, issues 9 and 10, volume 3, issues 6 and 7, and volume 4, issues 3 and 4, were published as combined issues. Volume 4 only had six issues. Volume 2, issue 7, and the combined issues 6 and 7 of volume 3 were "New Years'" issues. Volume 3, issue 1, was a "Special Issue on Malaria." In December 1943, after volume 4, issue 6, was published, the journal ceased publication. Altogether it published four volumes and forty-two issues. This journal's organization was simple. The number of editors, consultants, and workers was rather small. Tian Xiaoshi 田小石, Zhang Huizhong 張慧中, Zhou Yanlin 周燕麟, Wei Tongqing 魏桐青, Xue Zeshan 薛澤珊, Zhou Hongzhang 周紘章, Wei Xuan 魏萱, Li Zufang 李祖芳, and Wang Jiquan participated in the editing at various times.

The editor-in-chief, Tong Demao (1912–2002) was from Zhili Fangshan (now within the boundaries of the Beijing metropolitan area). His younger brother became ill and was harmed by an incompetent physician. He therefore became determined to study medicine. As a youth, he studied with Zhao Yanyuan 趙延元. In 1937, he graduated from the Chinese medicine department of North China National Medicine College (*Huabei guoyi xueyuan* 華北國醫學院) and worked in the clinic of the college president, Shi Jinmo 施今墨, for five years, obtaining Mr. Shi's true transmission of his skills and knowledge. In 1941, he opened a private clinic to benefit society. He, Wei Longxiang 魏龍驤, and two others, were known as "the four famous young physicians of Beijing." At various times, he was vice-president and head of general affairs at North China National Medicine College. The Chinese medical journals that he founded and edited include, *Chinese Medicine Monthly*, *Chinese Medicine Magazine*

© KONINKLIJKE BRILL NV, LEIDEN, 2020 | DOI:10.1163/9789004420724_043

(*Zhonghua yixue zazhi* 中華醫學雜誌), and *Beijing Chinese Medicine Monthly* (*Beijing zhongyi yuekan* 北京中醫月刊). He was both the society's president and the editor-in-chief. After the founding of the People's Republic, he became an assistant attending physician of internal medicine at the Guang'anmen hospital of the Health Ministry's Chinese Medical Research Institute (*Weisheng bu zhongyi yanjiu guang'anmen yiyuan* 衛生部中醫研究院廣安門醫院), assistant editor-in-chief and then editor-in-chief for *Chinese Medicine Magazine* (*Zhongyi zazhi* 中醫雜誌), a director for the Chinese Medicine Association (*Zhonghua yixue hui* 中華醫學會), and a member of the standing board of directors for the Chinese National Chinese Medicine Association (*Zhonghua quanguo zhongyi xuehui* 中華全國中醫學會).

In the 1930s and 40s the assault suffered by Chinese medicine at the hands of the development of modern medicine grew ever more severe. Chinese medicine was also suffering from unprecedented opposition and suppression. In 1937, in order to "develop culture and research national medical knowledge," Shi Jinmo, Zhou Jieren 周介人, and Lu Yuanlei founded the Beijing Chinese Medicine Society, all of the activities of which were later supported by Tong Demao. One year after the society was founded, they set about preparing for the founding of *Chinese Medicine Monthly*. They decided to "publish this journal as a field for the publication of society member's medical research" ("An Important Notice from the Beijing Chinese Medicine Society [*Beijing zhongyi xueshe jinyao qishi* 北京中醫學社緊要啟事]," volume 1, issue 3), so that together with like-minded people, they could "work together, rejecting the concept of lineage so that our knowledge can progress. We will not remain mired in Chinese medicine's strengths nor shield its deficiencies. We will use scientific methods to search for the true principles behind treatments. We will not be bound by the techniques of the past but will cast away its dross and preserve its essence, expunge its empty words and hasten toward practical application, causing the practice of our country's native medicine to join the ranks of the international medical community and thereby developing our Eastern culture" (Tong Demai, "*Chinese Medical Monthly*'s Declaration of Purpose [*Zhonguo yiyao yuekan chuangkan xuanyan* 中國醫藥月刊創刊宣言]," volume 1, issue 1).

For this journal's first two volumes, the journal's title was written by the famous physicians Shi Jinmo, Hou Yuwen 侯毓汶, and Fu Ruqin 傅汝勤. In the first two volumes there was a clear division between the columns. Starting with volume 1, issue 6, the table of contents on the cover contains a clear indication of the divisions that is obvious at a glance. In the third (with the exception of issue 11) and forth volumes, although there is no clear indication, judging by the content of the articles, the columns remained similar to the first two volumes. For the instruction of later students and the commending of former worthies, from volume 3, issue 1, onward, the left side of the cover successively published a brief biography, scholarly accomplishments, and photo of sixteen contemporary famous physicians: Shi Jinmo, Su Longyou 蕭龍友, Lu Yuanlei, Kong Bohua 孔伯華, Ding Zhongying 丁忠英, Zhang Cigong, Zhao Shuping 趙樹屏, Wang Fengchun 汪逢春, Liu Xingyuan 劉星垣, Song Daren 宋大仁, Zhang Juying 章巨膺, Yu Wuyan 余無言, Zhu Xiaonan 朱小南, Fan Tiantu 樊天徒, Ding Fubao 丁副保, and Mou Mingze 繆銘澤. It is a valuable historical resource on modern Chinese medical history.

43. Chinese Medicine (Zhongguo yixue 中國醫學)

In January 1941, *Chinese Medicine* was founded in Shanghai. Zhu Hegao 朱鶴皋 was the society president, and Shen Xinru 盛心如 was the editor-in-chief. They invited thirty-three people—including Ding Zhongyin 丁忠英, Yu Wuyan 余無言, Shi Yiren 時逸人, Zhu Weiju 祝味菊, Qin Bowei 秦伯未, and Cheng Menxue 程門雪—to be directors. They also invited forty-four people—including Wang Runmin 王潤民, You Xuezhou 尤學周, and Zhu Renkang 朱仁康—to be special contributors. This was a monthly journal, published on the fifteenth of every month. In March of the same year, it ceased publication, having published three issues in total.

The Chinese Medicine Magazine Society's guiding principles were, "to develop the local culture of Chinese medicine, to increase the people's health, and to bring together the two medical communities to strive to complete the mission of improving scholarship" ("Regulations of the Branch of Chinese Medicine Magazine Society [*Zhongguo yixue zazhi she fenshe jianzhang* 中國醫學雜誌社分社簡章]," issue 2). This society was based in Shanghai, but encouraged the formation of branch societies throughout the country. Its approach to running the journal was, "do foundational work in this period when there is panic over the subsistence of Chinese medical knowledge" ("Editor's Note [*Bianzhe de hua* 編者的話]," issue 1). They hoped to make the journal a bond by which to bring the dejected youth of the Chinese medicine community together to take up the important work before them—namely, the reviving of Chinese medicine.

The society's president, Zhu Hegao (1903–1995), was from Nantong, Jiangsu. He was the second son of Zhu Nanshan 朱南山. As a youth, he studied medicine with his father. In 1939, he became president of Shanghai Broad Kindness Chinese Medicine Hospital (*Shanghai guang'en zhongyiyuan* 上海廣恩中醫院). After 1946, he was a member of the Chinese Medicine Examination Committee of the Communist Government's Examination Institute (*Guomindang zhengfu kaoshi yuan zhongyi kaoshi weiyuan* 國民黨政府考試院中醫考試委員). After 1949, he moved to Hong Kong and was president of the Hong Kong New China Chinese Medicine Association (*Xianggang Xinhua zhongyi yixuehui* 香港新華中醫醫學會) and president of Hong Kong College of Chinese Medicine (*Xianggang zhongyi yixueyuan* 香港中醫醫學院). Later on, he was a medical consultant for Shanghai College of Chinese Medicine (*Shanghai zhongyi xueyuan* 上海中醫學院) and a consultant for the Hong Kong New China Association for the Advancement of Chinese Medicine and Medicinals

© KONINKLIJKE BRILL NV, LEIDEN, 2020 | DOI:10.1163/9789004420724_044

(*Xianggang Xinhua zhongyi zhongyao cujin hui* 香港新華中醫中藥促進會) as well as a committee member at the Sixth National Political Consultative Conference. Zhu Hegao's achievements in internal medicine were profound, and he was particularly skilled in gynecology. He was rigorous and precise in writing formulae but bold in his use of medicinals, and on occasion he innovated a new approach. His writings include *Essence of Treatment* (*Zhengzhi jinghua* 症治精華), *Teaching Materials on the Scientization of Chinese Medicine* (*Zhongyi kexuehua jiangyi* 中醫科學化講義), and *Mr. Zhu's Gynecology* (*Zhushi nüke* 朱氏女科).

The editor-in-chief, Sheng Xinru 盛心如 (1897–1954), used the courtesy name Shou'en 守恩 and the sobriquet "Disciple of Lanling Liquor." He was from Wujin, Jiangsu. From his childhood he was surpassingly intelligent. Through introductions from his family and friends, he was accepted as a student by the famous Shanghai physician Xue Wenyuan 薛文元 and studied assiduously, completely obtaining Mr. Xue's teaching. He was praised by Mr. Xue as his "most satisfactory student." After Mr. completed his studies, he ran a private clinic in Shanghai for more than thirty years, participating in the Shanghai's charitable organizations and the medical affairs of all of the factories. He was particularly skilled in treating internal medicine and gynecological illnesses as well as difficult and confusing syndromes. He, and the famous Shanghai physician, Cheng Menxue 稱門雪, were called "the two outstanding gentlemen by the sea (*haishang erjie* 海上二杰)." That was the period in which the Chinese medicine was the target of the Nationalist government's discrimination. Moreover, since "scholars scorn one another (*wenren xiangqing* 文人相輕)" many physicians were not willing to transmit their knowledge, but those famous Shanghai physicians, Cheng Menxue and Sheng Xinru, enjoyed resolving the perplexity and difficulties of young students. They were lauded as "the physicians of physicians." Sheng Xinru accepted employment at the Chinese Medical College (*Zhongguo yixueyuan* 中國醫學院), Chinese Medicine National Medical University (*Zhongyi guoyi daxue* 中醫國醫大學), Shanghai National Medicine Training Institute (*Shanghai guoyi zhuanxiu guan* 上海國醫專修館), and the New Chinese Medical College (*Xin Zhongguo yixueyuan* 新中國醫學院). He taught foundations of Chinese medicine and clinical practice. Mr. Sheng had innovative ideas about Chinese medicinals. His writings include *The Practical Study of Formulae* (*Shiyong fangji xue* 實用方劑學), *Gynecology* (*Fuke xue* 婦科學), *Prescribing* (*Chufang xue* 處方學), *Pediatrics* (*Erke xue* 兒科學), and *Warm Diseases* (*Wenbing xue* 溫病學).

The turning point for this journal was the unpopularity of the "Proposal to Abolish Chinese Medicine." Chinese medicine once again received the esteem of the country's people and particularly of the government authorities. The Education Ministry agreed to establish Chinese medicine training schools and to issue an outline Chinese medicine curriculum. Shi Yiren 時逸人, in his "The Process by which the Education Ministry Publicly Issued the Chinese Medicine Curriculum," pointed out, "In examining Chinese medicine, for a while they wanted to discard it from the educational system. Among the learned gentlemen of the Chinese medical community, there was not one who was not angry and concerned about this. It must be that medicine of Europe that invaded our country has already become a celebrated treasure and seized the place of the master. Now, fortunately, the Chinese medicine committee of the Health Bureau has joined with the medical education committee of the Education Ministry to form a Chinese Medicine Education Society (*Zhongguo yixue jiaoyu she* 中國醫學教育社) and that society has formulated an outline of the regulations for registering schools of Chinese medicine. With the acceptance of Minister Chen of the Education Ministry, those regulations have been publicly issued and enacted. From now on, the development of Chinese medicine can be counted on with certainty" (issue 1). This was the result of the fierce struggle of the members of the Chinese medical community.

In this journal's "Introduction (*Fakanci* 發刊詞)" it states, "Knowledge is the shared property of all under heaven. Medicine is that on which depends the strength or weakness of the country's people." However, owing to "self-centeredly hording secrets" and "the ideas of Buddhism, Daoism, and the school of the five phases getting mixed into medical theory," Chinese medicine "although it has four thousand years of history, is not as excellent as it was two thousand years ago." "If we do not progress we will regress. It is only common sense that one can anticipate the future by studying the past. There is wheel-rut one can follow." He called on the country's people who generally did not want to abolish Chinese medicine to embrace "the idea that knowledge is public (issue 1) and the need to work together to develop a thorough understanding, taking the strong points to supplement the weak points, discarding the dross and keep the essence, in order to develop Chinese medicine."

44. Chinese Women Physicians (Zhongguo nüyi 中國女醫)

In January 1941 (the thirtieth year of the Republican period), *Chinese Women Physicians* was founded in Shanghai by the president of the Society of Chinese Women Physicians (*Zhongguo nüyi xueshe* 中國女醫學社), Qian Baohua 錢寶華. Shanghai National Medicine Book Press (*Shanghai guoyi sushu ju* 上海國藥素書局) oversaw its publishing. Zhang Jingxia 張靜霞 was the editor-in-chief, and the other editors and important contributors included Gao Jianru 高鑒如, Zhang Jiayin 張嘉因, and Guo Duanlin 郭端麟. *Chinese Women Physicians* was originally a monthly periodical, coming out in the middle ten days of every month. In June, the fifth and sixth issues were published together. In July, the seventh and eighth issues were published together. Afterwards, the journal ceased publication, having published altogether eight issues.

The society president, Qian Baohua, was from Wujin, Jiangsu, and was born in a family of hereditary Chinese physicians. Her medical knowledge was learned from her father, Qian Tongzeng 錢同增 and uncle Qian Tonggao 錢同高 as well as her own efforts. She was particularly strong at gynecology and pediatrics. In the early years of the Republican period, she opened a clinic and saw patients, developing a strong reputation. Apart from clinical work, she was accustomed to promote and assist the Chinese medical profession. The editor-in-chief, Zhang Jingxia, was also a rather famous female Chinese medical physician. She was a student of Qian Tonggao, and classmate of Qian Baohua. She thoroughly studied gynecology and pediatrics, principally undertaking research and writing on Chinese medical theory.

Since the Republican period, the number of women Chinese physicians has gradually increased. Their signboards are frequently seen on the street, and they consistently participate in social activities as individuals. The unification of the entire community of female Chinese medical doctors, however, has yet to occur. *Chinese Women Physicians* was founded on the principles of "… promoting the spirit of mutual aid among the entire community of women physicians, struggling together, developing each female physician's theoretical consciousness, and mutual encouragement." It was founded to develop and promote the profession of Chinese women physicians. After publishing two issues it received the accolades, "opening a new path for national medicine's female community and increasing the splendor of China's scholarship," "unprecedentedly well-qualified, opening a new chapter in the Republic's medical history," and "the content is rich and abundant and the arguments brilliant." Qin Bowei wrote an article offering advice on achieving the journal's aspirations. Zhu Hegao 朱鶴皋 also declared that Qian Baohua was "the ideal female physician." From all of this we can see the interest the Chinese medical world felt regarding *Chinese Women Physicians*.

Chinese Women Physicians was devoted to developing and improving the knowledge of female Chinese medical physicians. It provided a platform for community and communication among women Chinese medical physicians. It improved their social status, expanded their social influence, and contributed to the transmission of theoretical knowledge and clinical experience within the community of female Chinese medical doctors.

45. Medical Literature (Yiwen 醫文)

On April 15th, 1943 (the thirty-second year of the Republican period), *Medical Literature* was founded in Shanghai by the famous Chinese medical historian of that time, Fan Xingzhun 范行準. Laiqingge Bookhouse (*Laiqingge shuzhuang* 來青閣書莊) acted as his agent. It was a monthly journal and altogether published six issues.

The editor-in-chief and publisher, Fan Xingzhun (1906–1998) was named Di 適 and used the courtesy name Tianqing 天聲. He was from Tangxi Houda village, Zhejiang. When he was young, he was extremely poor. From the age of thirteen he worked as a student in the medicinal store opened by his uncle. At the age of sixteen he completed his apprenticeship. At the age of eighteen he returned to his village and intensively studied Chinese medicine for two years. At the age of twenty, he began practicing medicine in his village, which he continued to do for three years. Afterwards he entered the Shanghai National Medical College (*Shanghai guoyi xueyuan* 上海國藥學院). After completing his studies, he practiced medicine in Shanghai working for the Shanghai Chinese Medicine Association (*Shanghai zhonghua yixue hui* 上海中華醫學會), the Chinese Medicine Magazine Society (*Zhonghua yixue zazhi she* 中華醫學雜誌社), and the Chinese-Western Medical Research Society (*Zhong-xi yiyao yanjiu she* 中西醫藥研究社). He undertook research on medical history as well as editorial work for the medical journals, *Chinese Medicine Magazine* (*Zhonghua yixue zazhi* 中華醫學雜誌) and the *Medical History Magazine* (*Yishi zazhi* 醫史雜誌). His writings include *Medical Knowledge Transmitted from the West during the Ming* (*Mingji xiyang chuanru yixue* 明季西洋傳入醫學), *An Intellectual History of Chinese Preventative Medicine* (*Zhongguo yufang yixue sixiangshi* 中國預防醫學思想史), *An Outline of Chinese Medical History* (*Zhongguo yixue shilue* 中國醫學史略), and *New Ideas on the History of Disease in China* (*Zhongguo bingshi xinyi* 中國病史新義). He is one of the most famous medical historian and bibliographer of modern and contemporary China.

This journal's cover was succinct and clear. It displayed the two characters "醫文" ("Medical Literature") written in intaglio in China's traditional seal-carving script. Thick and heavy without losing its attractiveness, it showed that Chinese medical culture is firm like the base and broad foundations of a huge rock. From the fifth issue onward, the table of contents included not only the titles, authors, and page numbers of the articles, but also clearly indicated basic information about the journal including its place of publication, its sites of distribution, the location and price of advertisements, and notes on advertisements.

© KONINKLIJKE BRILL NV, LEIDEN, 2020 | DOI:10.1163/9789004420724_046

46. New China Medicine Monthly (Xin Zhonghua yiyao yuekan 新中華醫藥月刊)

In February 1945 (the thirty-fourth year of the Republican period), Shen Yannan 沈炎南, Gao Deming 高德明，Hu Guangci 胡光慈, Li Rupeng 李汝鵬, and Wang Fumin 王福民 founded *New China Medicine Monthly* in Chongqing. The president of the society and publisher of the journal was Shen Yannan. Gao Deming and Hu Guanci were the managers. The society's headquarters were located at #17, Linhua Street, Guanyin Yan, Chongqing. The journal was published on the twenty-fifth of every month (on occasion two issues were published together). After more than two years, the journal published its last issue on May 25th, 1947, having published a total of three volumes and twenty-seven issues.

The founders of the journal were among the well-known physicians of the time. The society president and publisher of the journal, Shen Yannan, was a famous physician of Chonqing at the time. He had been a member of the Central National Medicine Institute's editorial committee and chair of the New China Medicine Association's tuberculosis committee. The editor-in-chief, Gao Deming, was at various times a member of the Health Office's Chinese medicine committee, a member of the Education Ministry's Chinese medicine professional education committee, vice-president of the National Secondary Capital Chinese Medicine Hospital (*Guoli peidu zhongyi yuan* 國立陪都中醫院), a consultant for the Logistics Department of the Rear, a member of the Chinese medical doctor examination committee of the Ministry of Examinations, and a member of the medical personal examination committee. The editor-in-chief, Hu Guangci, had, at various times, been a member of the Health Office's Chinese medicine committee, a member of the Education Ministry's Chinese medicine professional education committee, and director of the department of pediatrics at the National Secondary Capital Chinese Medicine Hospital. Wang Fumin was successively a member of the Central National Medicine Institute's editorial committee, an attending physician in the National Secondary Capital Chinese Medicine Hospital's gynecology department, and vice-president of the Health Ministry's Secondary Capital Chinese Medicine Hospital. Each of them made a contribution to the Chinese medical community and held a high position governmentally and academically. For that reason, the papers they wrote were guaranteed to arouse interest at the time and exert a considerable social influence.

© KONINKLIJKE BRILL NV, LEIDEN, 2020 | DOI:10.1163/9789004420724_047

47. West China Medical Magazine (Huaxi yiyao zazhi 華西醫藥雜誌)

On April 15th, 1946 (the thirty-fifth year of the Republican period), *West China Medical Magazine* was founded in Chongqing by the president and general manager of the Chinese-Western Medical Publication Society (*Zhong-Xi yiyao tushu she* 中西醫藥圖書社), Zhou Fusheng 周復生. It was published and printed by the Chinese-Western Medical Publication Society. Lu Yuanlei 陸淵雷 wrote the title for the journal in his calligraphy. This journal invited Ren Yingqiu 任應秋 and Wang Jiequan 汪洁權 to be editors-in-chief and seventeen people, including Jiang Chunhua 姜春華 and Ye Juquan 葉橘泉, to be part of the editorial committee. Zhang Jueren 張覺人 managed distribution in Chengdu. They invited twenty-six people—including Shi Jinmo 時今墨, Chen Cunren 陳存仁, Qin Bowei 秦伯未, Zhang Zanchen 張贊臣, and Wu Zhaoxian 吳棹仙—to act as consultants. They also invited sixty-six people—including Lu Yuanlei, Zhang Cigong 張次公, Ye Juquan, Zhang Juying 張巨膺, Jiang Chunhua, Zhu Liangchun 朱良春, Qiu Peiran 裘沛然, and Jiang Zuojing 姜佐景—to be special contributors. They initially planned for it to be a monthly journal, with a complete year of twelve issues constituting one volume. In actual operation, however, there were some adjustments.

The first volume was published monthly, but in the second volume it was alternately a published monthly and bimonthly. For the third volume, it changed to become a seasonal publication before finally ceasing publication altogether. After the founding of the New China, this journal published a single special issue, but failed to continue operation afterwards.

After the Chinese-Western Medical Publication Society began operation, it not only edited, published, and distributed *West China Medical Magazine*, but also continued to publish opening announcements for private practices on the journal's back cover. At the same time, for the readers of its publications, this book society procured high quality paper and published "almost two hundred essential Chinese and Western medical publications, on topics ranging from the *Treatise on Cold Damage*, *Essentials of the Golden Coffer*, and warm-heat diseases to modern internal medicine, diagnosis, pathology, and medicinals. It has searched for and brought together many books, soliciting reading material for our readers and distributing old books." This led to this book society possessing many services for readers, such as editing and publishing as well as supplying documents and books.

© KONINKLIJKE BRILL NV, LEIDEN, 2020 | DOI:10.1163/9789004420724_048

Ren Yingqiu (1914–1984) used the courtesy name Hongbin 鴻濱. He was from Jiangjin Youxi, Sichuan (part of modern Chongqing). He was a famous contemporary Chinese medical physician and educator. He was born into a family of scholar-physicians. From his childhood, he adored the classics and medical texts. He had a rather solid foundation in the classics, history, and ancient Chinese philosophy. At the age of seventeen, he began studying the Chinese medical classics with the famous local physician of the times, Liu Youyu 劉有餘 while also establishing the Benefit the World Clinic (*Jishi zhenmaisuo* 濟世診脈所). In 1936, he went to study at the Shanghai Chinese Medical College (*Shanghai Zhongguo yixueyuan* 上海中國醫學院), where he had the opportunity to request instruction from the famous Shanghai physicians of the day, including Ding Zhongyin 丁忠英, Xie Liheng 謝利恆, Cao Yingfu 曹穎甫, Lu Yuanlei 陸淵雷, Zhuang Wenfang 莊文芳, Guo Bailiang 郭柏良, and Wu Keqian 吳克潛. His outlook broadened with each passing day and he made great strides in his studies. Following the Japanese invasion, he broke off his studies in Shanghai and returned to Sichuan to practice medicine and begin writing books and developing theories. It was the first sign of his prodigious abilities. Prior to 1954, he emphasized the scientization of Chinese medicine. Afterwards, he devoted his energies to the work of unearthing and organizing Chinese medical theory. After the Liberation, he taught at Chongqing Chinese Medical School (*Chongqing zhongyi xuexiao* 重慶中醫學校). In 1957, he moved to Beijing Chinese Medical School (*Beijing zhongyi xuexiao* 北京中醫學校).

Wang Jiequan's dates are unclear. He used the courtesy name Shenzhi 慎之 and was from Shanghai. He was a student of the famous modern physician, Zhang Cigong 章次公. He was the editor of *A New Voice on National Medicine* and *A Collection of Proven Formulae* (*Yanfang jicheng* 驗方集成) as well as an editor and important contributor to *Chinese Medicine Monthly*. His writings include "A Selection of Chinese Medical Treatises (*Zhongguo yiyao lunwen xuan* 中國醫藥論文選)" (January, 1949), "Treating Bacillary and Amebic Dysentery with Single Medicinals (*Dui ganjun liji ji amiba liji de danwei yao zhiliao* 對桿菌痢疾及阿米巴痢疾的單味藥治療)" (*Chinese Medicine Magazine* [*Zhongyi zazhi* 中醫雜誌], 1955, issue 8), and "The Motherland's Medicine's Understanding and Treatment of Infectious Hepatitis (*Zuguo yixue dui chuanranxing ganyan de renshi he zhiliao* 祖國醫學對傳染性肝炎的認識和治療)" (*Liaoning Chinese Medicine Magazine* [*Liaoning zhongyi zazhi* 遼寧中醫雜誌], 1960, issue 3).

48. Medical History Magazine (Yishi zazhi 醫史雜誌)

In March 1947 (the thirty-sixth year of the Republican period), *Medical History Magazine* was founded in Shanghai. This journal was a seasonal publication in the 16mo printing format, published in bilingually in Chinese and English. The number of pages in each issue was not fixed. During the Republican period, it published a total of two volumes and eight issues. It was edited and published by the *Medical History Magazine* editorial committee of the Chinese Medical History Association (*Zhonghua yishi xuehui* 中華醫史學會). The editor-in-chief was Yu Yan 余岩. The manager-in-chief was Wang Jimin 王吉民.

In the autumn of 1935, at the Third Plenary Conference of the Chinese Medicine Association (*Zhonghua yixuehui* 中華醫學會) in Guangzhou, Wang Jimin, Wu Liande 伍連德, Yi Bo'en 伊博恩 (B.E. Read), Hu Mei 胡美 (E.H. Hume), Li Yousong 李友松, Hai Shende 海深德 (L.S. Huizenga), and Yang Jishi 楊濟時 "Reflected on the fact that the long history of our country's medicine contains riches that are in need of organization and research, but there was not yet an organization carrying out this work." They therefore formed the medical history committee (see Wang Jimin, "A Report on the Work of this Association over the Last Ten Years [*Shinian lai benhui gongzuo baogao* 十年來本會工作報告]," volume 1, issue 1). At that time, Wang Jimin was elected as chair. Yi Bo'en was the secretary, and Li Yousong, Yang Jishi, and Hu Mei were committee members. In February 1936, with the consent of the board of directors of the Chinese Medicine Association, the medical history committee was formally established. In 1937, at the Fourth Plenary Conference of the Chinese Medicine Association in Shanghai, the medical history committee was formed anew with expanded scope. Its name was changed to the Chinese Medical History Association, and Wang Jimin became president. The Chinese Medical History Association is one of the earliest branch specialty associations established by the Chinese Medicine Association. After the establishment of the Chinese Medical History Association, the outline of the association's work was decided upon. It included searching for and collecting texts related to medical history, publishing *Medical History Magazine*, translating the Chinese medical classics, printing and publicizing the research achievements of the association members, establishing a Chinese medical library, and founding a medical history museum. Due to financial difficulties and the outbreak of the Pacific War, from 1936 to 1947, The Medical History Association of the Chinese Medicine Association made use of *Chinese Medicine Magazine*

© KONINKLIJKE BRILL NV, LEIDEN, 2020 | DOI:10.1163/9789004420724_049

(*Zhonghua yixue zazhi* 中華醫學雜誌) to publish one special medical history issue each year. Altogether, they published nine issues in this fashion—five in Cheese, four in English. They also published an anniversary issue on the fifth anniversary of the establishment of the Chinese Medical History Association. It contained fifteen specialist articles in Chinese and English. After victory was obtained in the War of Resistance,[1] reflecting on the fact that "The association's members are spread across the country and internationally—already including citizens of more than seven countries. The distance between members is already broad and everyone is suffering from the difficulty of communications. Moreover, everyone's work is also suffering from the lack of a place to publish it. If we wish to facilitate our learning from each other, comparisons between Chinese and foreign medical history, urgently needed mutual translations, and overcoming our own deficiencies by learning from others, how can we advocate for this if we don't have a written record?" ("Introduction [*Fakanci* 發刊詞]," volume 1, issue 1). In the winter of 1946, the yearly conference of the Chinese Medical History Association agreed to publish *Medical History Magazine* and make it the mouthpiece of the organization, in order to "publish translations by researchers on the medical history of China and foreign countries as our primary aim" ("Notice to Contributors [*Gaoyue* 稿約]," volume 1, issue 1). They then formed the editorial committee to handle the work of the journal. At the first meeting of the editorial committee, Yu Yan was the chair and Wang Jimin was the manager. The committee included Yi Bo'en, Li Yousong, and Fan Xingzhun 范行準. The founding of *Medical History Magazine* coincided with the tenth anniversary of the Chinese Medical History Association. The first issue was a tenth anniversary commemorative publication. From this time onward, our country had a magazine devoted to medical history. It was also our country's earliest specialized medical history publication.

Medical History Magazine's editor-in-chief, Yu Yan (1879–1954) used the sobriquet Baizhi 百之 and the courtesy name Yunxiu 雲岫. He went by his courtesy name. He was a modern physician from Zhenyuyancun, Xiepu, Zhenhai, Zhejiang. In 1884, at the age of six, he entered a private village school. In 1901, he began studying in Nanxun's Nanxunxi Public School (*Nanxunxi gongxue* 南潯溪公學). In 1903, he moved to Shanghai and became a teacher at Chengzhong School (*Chengzhong xuetang* 澄衷學堂). In 1905, he was recommended by Zhenhai Kunchi Academy (*Zhenhai kunchi shuyuan* 鎮海昆池書院) and moved to japan to study on a public scholarship. In 1908, he entered Japan's Ōsaka Medical University's (*Ōsaka ika daigaku* 大阪醫科大學) preparatory

---

studies department. In 1911, the 1911 Revolution broke out, and he returned to China to take part in the revolutionary army's relief work. He raced about Shaanxi and other places energetically serving the people on behalf of the revolutionary army. In the spring of 1913, he returned to Japan's Ōsaka Medical University to continue his studies. He graduated in 1916. After returning to China, he became the head of medical affairs for Shanghai Hospital (*Shanghai yiyuan* 上海醫院). The following year he resigned. In 1918, he opened a clinic in Shanghai while also becoming an editor for the Shanghai Commercial Press (*Shanghai shangwu yinshuguan* 上海商務印書館). In 1928, he founded the weekly publication, *Social Medicine Journal* (*Shehui yibao* 社會醫報). Yu Yan had researched a bit about Chinese medicine and Chinese medicinals. He had definite attainments in the exegesis and textual criticism of ancient Chinese medical texts. His *Explicating the Meaning of the Names and Indications of Ancient Diseases* (*Gudai jibing minghou shuyi* 古代疾病名候疏義) examined the origin and development of ancient concepts of disease and is an aid to research into ancient diseases. Since he had been influenced by Japanese Meiji reforms' ban of Kampō medicine (*Kanpō igaku* 漢方醫學), he thought that Chinese medical theory was "unscientific" and Chinese medicine needed a "revolution." Because of this he emphasized "abolishing the medicine but retaining the medicinals" and in 1929, at the first meeting of the Central Health Committee (*Zhongyang weisheng weiyuanhui* 中央衛生委員會) held by the Nanjing government's Health Ministry, submitted "A Proposal for Abolishing Old Medicine in order to Clear away Obstacles to Medicine and Health (*Feizhi jiuyi yi saochu yishi weisheng zhang'ai an* 廢止舊醫以掃除醫事衛生之障礙案)," which was accepted. It was a great setback in the history of the development of Chinese medicine at that time, but it could not be enforced due to the stringent opposition of the Chinese medical community. Mr. Yu was at various times the president of the Shanghai Physician's Trade Association (*Shanghai yishi gonghui* 上海醫師公會), a member of the special committee on health of the Nanjing government's Ministry of the Interior, a consultant for the medical education committee (*Yixue jiaoyu weiyuanhui* 醫學教育委員會), and president of the Chinese Medical Research Institute (*Zhongguo yiyao yanjiusuo* 中國醫藥研究所). After the founding of the New China, he was successively a member of special committee on Chinese medicine of the national health science research committee (*quanguo weisheng kexue yanjiu weiyuanhui zhongyi zhuanmen weiyuanhui* 全國衛生科學研究委員會中醫專門委員會), a member of the federation of the Chinese natural sciences special committee (*Zhonghua ziran kexue zhuanmen hui lianhehui* 中華自然科學專門會聯合會), and a director of the Chinese Medicine Association. Apart from *Explicating the Meaning of the Names and Indications of Ancient Diseases*, his writings include *A Treatise on Medical Revolution* (*Yixue geming lun* 醫學革命論), *A Continuation of the Treatise on Medical Revolution* (*Yixue geming lun xuji* 醫學革命論續集), and *Deliberations on the Numinous Pivot and Basic Questions*[2] (*Lingsu shangdui* 靈素商兌).

Medical History Magazine's manager-in-chief, Wang Jimin (1889–1972), used the courtesy name Jiaxiang 嘉祥 and sobriquet Yunxin 芸心. He was from Dongguan, Guangdong. In 1910, he graduated from Hong Kong Western Medicine University (*Xianggang xiyi daxuetang* 香港西醫大學堂). He was president of the Chinese Epidemic Prevention Medical Institute (*Zhongguo fangyi yiyuan* 中國防疫醫院) among other posts. In 1937, he accepted an invitation to come to Shanghai to assist in the management of the affairs of the Chinese Medicine Association. He was also elected as the vice-president of the Chinese Medicine Association. He was a modern pioneer in researching our country's medical history. He noticed that the American medical historian, Fielding Hudson Garrison's, *An Introduction to the History of Medicine*[3] made little mention of medical historical materials from our country and contained many errors relating to it. He then resolved to collect materials for a history of Chinese medicine. He devoted himself to the research and, together with Dr. Wu Liande 伍連德, wrote the first part of an English publication on Chinese medical history, *The History of Chinese Medicine* (*Zhongguo yishi* 中國醫史), published in 1932. It created a deep impression on the international medical history community. In 1935, he sponsored the establishing of the medical history committee of the Chinese Medicine Association and was elected its chair. In 1937, he made arrangements for a medical history exposition at the Chinese Medicine Association. In 1938, our country's first medical history museum, the Chinese Medicine Association's Medical History Museum (*Zhonghua yixuehui yishi bowuguan* 中國醫學會博物館), was established and Wang Jimin was the museum's president. In 1959, this museum was incorporated into Shanghai College of Chinese Medicine (*Shanghai zhongyi xueyuan* 上海中醫學院), and Wang Jimin continued as its president. Mr. Wang was a medical history lecturer and assistant professor at the National Sino-French Medical College (*Guoli Zhong-Fa yixueyuan* 國立中法醫學院) and Shanghai College of Chinese Medicine. He was also the assistant editor-in-chief for

---

2   The *Numinous Pivot* (*Lingshu* 靈樞) and *Basic Questions* (*Suwen* 素問) are the two parts of the *Yellow Emperor's Inner Classic* (*Huangdi neijing* 黃帝內經), the foundational text of Chinese medicine.

3   The original text does not provide a translation of the name or title of this text, saying merely "嘉立林的《醫學史》." However, Garrison was an American and his book, published in 1913, was hailed as a landmark in the field, making it likely this is the author and text referred to.

Chinese Medicine Magazine (*Zhonghua yixue zazhi* 中華醫學雜誌). In June of 1949, he was made a corresponding member of the International History of Science Research Institute (*Guoji kexueshi yanjiuyuan* 國際科學史研究院). In October 1966, he was made a full member of the International History of Science Research Institute. Mr. Wang devoted his entire life to researching medical history, and he pursued his studies stringently. Apart from *The History of Chinese Medicine*, his writings include *Illuminating Medicine in Chinese History* (*Zhongguo lidai yixue zhi faming* 中國歷代醫學之發明), *An Index of Foreign Language Materials for Chinese Medical History* (*Zhongguo yishi waiwen wenxian suoyin* 中國醫史外文文獻索引), and *Examination of the Circulation of the Motherland's Medical Culture Overseas* (*Zuguo yiyao wenhua liuchuan haiwai kao* 祖國醫藥文化流傳海外考) as well as more than one hundred articles on medical history.

Appendix: A Humanist Analysis on Periodicals of Chinese Medicine from the Late Qing and Republican Periods

Twentieth-Century China, 40.1, 69–78, January 2015

Wang Youpeng
Shanghai Lexicographical Publishing House, China

Translated by David Luesink
University of Pittsburgh, USA
luesink@pitt.edu

Abstract

This article introduces English-language scholars to *The Compilation of Chinese Medicine Periodicals from the Late Qing and Republican Periods*, a valuable new scholarly resource edited by Wang Youpeng. Compilation projects like this one have been a major field of scholarship in China from imperial times and serve the purpose of both preserving and selecting texts from around the empire. The medical journals included in this compilation took advantage of the newly available technology of print capitalism in Shanghai to respond to the challenge posed by a rapidly organizing Western medicine that sought to regulate and abolish Chinese medical practitioners. This article is a translation of Wang Youpeng's introduction to *The Compilation* and was first published in the *China Reader's Journal* (Zhonghua dushu bao) in August 2012. Wang argues that Chinese medical journals of this period are one of the best sources for observing the changing nature of medical practice and education during the late Qing and Republican eras so crucial to the development of medicine and science in China. *The Compilation* is a massive primary source not only for understanding the modern transformation of Chinese medicine from a private to a public endeavor, but also the larger role of medicine in Chinese society, seen through published documents on the battle between proponents and enemies of Chinese medicine. Literature specialists will be interested in the many short stories on medicine by important Chinese writers like Bing Xin. Ultimately, Wang argues, *The Compilation* should stimulate a multitude of new research projects. Given its importance in bringing together these journals from repositories all over China, we might add that research libraries and specialists may consider acquiring this substantive source and the separate index and abstracted table of contents.

Keywords

Chinese medicine – periodicals – late Qing and Republican periods

The Compilation of Chinese Medicine Periodicals from the Late Qing and Republican Periods (中国近代中医药期刊汇编 *Zhongguo jindai zhongyiyao qikan huibian*, hereafter *The Compilation*) altogether has 212 sections and was jointly published by Shanghai University of Traditional Chinese Medicine and Shanghai Lexicographical Publishing House in 2012 (上海中医药大学 Shanghai zhongyiyao daxue and 上海辞书出版社 Shanghai cishu chubanshe). The chance to edit this book came out of a fortuitous conversation that Duan Yishan (段逸山 b. 1940) and I had one evening in a conference hotel in Beijing. Duan, a tenured professor at Shanghai University of Traditional Chinese Medicine, and at that time also the head of the library, was then directing several doctoral students to research late Qing and Republican era Chinese medicine periodicals. There were few people doing research on these journals, and the Shanghai University of Traditional Chinese Medicine had a particularly good collection, making this a treasure-house well deserving of increased scholarly attention. Professor Duan's introduction made me eager to do something immediately, so I began conceiving ideas of how to get this project started.

Science and technology periodicals from the late Qing and Republican eras are very numerous because of the rapid development of science and technology in China at the time, and for this reason they have been widely recognized as retaining historical value even to the present day. Periodicals from Chinese medicine have not been recognized as such, and yet they nonetheless should be considered as one type of science and technology periodical, possessing at least two kinds of value as historical documents. First, the medical conferences, medical cases, and effective prescriptions of a century ago have a very important contemporary reference value for both clinical Chinese medicine and research on pharmaceuticals—some prescriptions may still be able to be used clinically. But because even large libraries have rarely collected this type of periodical, a systematic collection and publication of the most important journals in one set could represent the development of the sequence of ideas of modern Chinese medicine, and this would have major academic significance for the study and continuation of Chinese medicine. On that particular evening, Duan and I talked very excitedly about all of this as our ideas came together, and we decided that, after returning to Shanghai, each of us would report to our supervisors with a list of items for the project. Not long after, under the direction of each of our supervisors and of the late Mr. Qiu Peiran (裘沛然 1916–2010), one of China's great physicians, Shanghai University of Traditional Chinese Medicine and Shanghai Lexicographical Publishing House established an editorial work team. Further, with the periodical collections of Shanghai University of Traditional Chinese Medicine Library, the Museum of Traditional Chinese Medicine, and the library of the Lexicographical Publishing House, we started an extended five-year process of compilation.

Many hundreds of medical and pharmaceutical periodicals were published in the late Qing and Republican periods, and among those more than two hundred relate to Chinese medicine. But many of this number were very short-lived, publishing only one or two issues before laying down the flag and stilling the drums. So the most important question became how to select periodicals for inclusion. Duan Yishan established five principles of selection: the first was to emphasize journals that focused on Chinese rather than Western medicine; second was to privilege journals with early publication dates, especially the most influential ones; third was to privilege those periodicals with a longer publication run; fourth was to privilege those that were relatively authoritative, or that had significant influence. These four principles guaranteed that *The Compilation* would collect all of the most important Chinese medicine periodicals of the late Qing and Republican periods. For example, from the Guangxu and Xuantong periods of the Qing Dynasty (1875–1911), *Report of the Academy of Beneficial Aid* (利济学堂报 *Liji xuetang bao*), *Medical News* (医学报 *Yixue bao*), *Shaoxing Medical Journal* (绍兴医药学报 *Shaoxing yiya-oxue bao*), *Chinese-Western Medical Journal* (中西医学报 *Zhong-Xi yixue bao*) and Shanxi's *Medical Magazine* (医学杂志 *Yixue zazhi*), *Annals of the Medical World* (医界春秋 *Yijie chunqiu*), and *Mainstay of National Medicine* (国医砥柱 *Guoyi dizhu*) were each published for more than ten years. Qiu Jisheng (裘吉生 1873–1947), head editor of *March Third Medical Journal*, He Lianchen (何廉臣 1861–1929), and Cao Bingzhang (曹炳章 1878–1956) founders of *Shaoxing Medical Monthly*, as well as Zhang Xichun (张锡纯 1860–1933) and Liu Jingsu (刘景素 dates unknown), head editors of *Shenyang Medical Journal*, and so on, all comprised a famous generation of Chinese physicians. As a fifth principle, unique medical journals with special interest were selected; for example, *Medical Literature*, *Chinese Women's Medicine*, and so on. The former is important for researching documents of medical history, while the latter is the only journal edited and published by female practitioners of Chinese medicine, and a medical periodical that was geared toward female practitioners of Chinese medicine as readers. According to these principles, 49 different periodicals were collected in five parts from Beijing, Tianjin, Shanxi, Shanghai, Suzhou, Shaoxing, Wenzhou, Guangzhou, Shenyang, and Hong Kong, each in order of their first publication date. The volumes became available in 2012.

On May 23, 2012, Shanghai University of Traditional Chinese Medicine and Shanghai Lexicographical Publishing House convened a publishing symposium in the Great Hall of the People in Beijing for *The Compilation of Chinese Medical Periodicals in the Late Qing and Republican Periods*. It was enthusiastically attended by many important officials, including Han Qide, National People's Assembly Vice Committee Head and chair of the Association of Chinese Scientists, Wu Shulin, Assistant Director of the News Publishing Administration, Wu Gang, Vice Bureau Chief of the National Traditional Chinese Medicine Management Office, and also by Chen Kaixian of the Chinese Academy of Sciences, Zhang Boli of the Chinese Academy of Engineers, and a total of close to 100 representatives congratulating us on the successful completion of this broad cultural undertaking and giving a full measure of affirmation to the project. The speeches of the leaders and professionals at the conference, the conversations before and after the conference, and the process of editing *The Compilation* over several years engendered some realizations for me that I would like to record and share.

1   A Richly Colored Historical Scroll

Chinese medicine has been a relatively conservative, self-contained scholarly domain. In order to protect the medical skills of a single family, historically Chinese medicine was like a religious discipline passed down to sons, but not to daughters, transmitted to daughters-in-law but not to sons-in-law. But when Chinese medical journals appeared in the late Qing and Republican periods, they broke open the quiet aspect of Chinese medicine's closed lines of transmission.

Chen Qiu (陈虬 1851–1904) Zhou Xueqiao (周雪樵 ?-1910), Wang Wenqiao (王问樵), He Lianchen, Qiu Jisheng, Ding Fubao (丁福保 1874–1952), and so on—this group of famous practitioners of Chinese medicine—one after another established China's first set of famous modern medical periodicals, and they used their journals to pass on medical skills, leading to an opening of the general mood of the medical world. Chen Qiu's famous medical publication "A Diagnostic Record of the Cottage of Stings" (蜇庐诊录 Zhe lu zhen lu) was printed in *Report of the Academy of Beneficial Aid*, recording the author's clinical evidential effectiveness. *Medical News* printed "Mr. Zhu Ya'nan's Medical Casebook" (朱雅 南先生医案 Zhu Ya'nan xiansheng yi'an) and "Xueqiao's

Medical Casebook" (雪　樵医案 Xueqiao yi'an) and solicited wide-ranging secret and proven prescriptions, to make them known to the public. *Shaoxing Medical Journal* called for individual reports from the Chinese medical world of knowledge gained from clinical experience, in order to make these medical cases known to the world. The 49 collected periodicals in *The Compilation* could be called an assembly of famous physicians, with innumerable schools presenting themselves. This exchange greatly invigorated the scholarly atmosphere of the Chinese medical world, and leaves a valuable medical inheritance for posterity.

At the beginning of the twentieth century, periodicals were rather like the internet today. This type of newly popular communication media developed swiftly and fiercely. The fact that the content of the new print media was abundant and diverse, and that it had the ability to report quickly, were both deeply welcomed by the scholarly world and by the reading public. Late Qing and Republican Chinese medical periodicals present to everyone not only news related to Chinese medicine, but also represent medical news of the moment, as well as news of all kinds of current politics and information about society and culture. The "Of Record" (报录 Baolu) column in the *Report of the Academy of Beneficial Aid* played a significant role in opening eyes to the world outside of China by transmitting new areas of study and encouraging reform. Examples of items include "Random News of Foreign Affairs" (洋务掇闻 Yangwu duo wen), "New Records of Scholarly Shade" (学部新录 Xue bu xin lu), "Trivial Words on Agricultural Studies" (农学琐言 Nongxue suo yan), "Unofficial Annals of Artistic/ Skillful Matters" (艺事稗乘 Yishi bai sheng), "Collected Writings on Commerce" (商务丛谈 Shangwu congtan), "External Annals of Beneficial Aid" (利济外乘 Liji wai sheng), "Vessel of the Sayings of Natural Science" (格致卮言 Gezhi zhi yan), "Notes on Contemporary Politics" (近政备考 Jin zheng beikao), "Literary Writings on Statecraft" (经世文传 Jingshi wen zhuan), "Contemporary Information" (见闻近录 Jian wen jin lu), and so on, quoting from more than 30 different Chinese newspapers and more than 20 foreign-language newspapers. And so the very format of the journals reflects the kaleidoscope of society.

Scholars have identified China's very first periodical as *Wu's Medical Talks Collectanea* (吴医汇讲 Wu yi hui jiang) from the seventeenth year of the Qianlong reign (1792), and its content and form can already be said to be basically a prototype of a journal. But this was only a random occurrence in history, and at that time it did not spawn a new media form. *The Compilation* takes *Report of the Academy of Beneficial Aid* as the fountainhead of Chinese medical periodicals, for although its format was still traditional, its publication cycle and content had already adapted completely to the demands of the newly developed media. The 49 journals that came after it for the next half-century were a true record of the era and together provide a detailed, vibrant historical scroll. By means of our hard work in bringing them together as *The Compilation*, readers can now conveniently encounter these journals as a single book, inspecting nearly half a century of social transformations and medical progress. This is truly the cultural power and social value embodied in the publication of large-scale collections like this one.

2   Thinking from the Debates between Chinese and Western Medicine

The value of the documents in these periodicals for researching Chinese medicine and drugs goes without saying, so I do not need to go into unnecessary detail about these here. But what jumps out at me with most power from these periodicals are humanist reflections on the arguments between Chinese and Western medicine. Periodicals are produced to be relevant to a very particular time, so major events are all first reflected there. For example, in 1935, Wang Jingwei (汪精卫 1883–1944), at that time the secretary of the Executive Branch of the National Government, wrote a letter to Sun Ke (孙科 1891–1973), secretary of the Legislative Branch, trying to block the proclamation of legislation on the Statutes on National Medicine. After Zhang Zanchen (张赞臣 1904–1993), editor of *Annals of the Medical World*, obtained "Wang Jingwei's Letter to Sun Ke" (汪精卫 致孙科书 Wang Jingwei zhi Sun Ke shu), he immediately took a photograph and made a printing plate, publishing it in issue 105, and wrote an article titled "Battle Cry and Attack" (鸣鼓而攻 Ming gu er gong) which became explosive news, located on the cover of the journal. The article ridiculed "the great Secretary of the Legislative Branch," Wang Jingwei, with biting satire that showed no mercy:

> Wang's college mistress skillfully brought a complaint while they lay in bed. As the darkness comes, so will the darkness leave. In the matter of issuing such obfuscation of private requests and selfish commitments, such terrible things must surely come to light.

Under the pressure of public opinion, the Statutes on National Medicine were finally made public.

In surveying the history of Chinese medical journals in this period—the convergence of Chinese and Western medicine, the scientificization of Chinese medicine, the movement to "abolish Chinese medicine, preserve Chinese drugs," the movement to "abolish Chinese medicine"—all of these are perennial subjects of conversation in this historical era. This type of dispute could also be called Chinese medicine's search to find a path forward. This process can be said to have originated with the late Qing scholar of national learning, Yu Yue (俞樾 1821–1907, *hao*: Qu Yuan 曲园), who for the first time offered opposition to the theory of Chinese medicine in *Treatise on Abolishing Medicine* (废医论 *Fei yi lun*) and *Treatise on Medical Care and Medicines* (医药论 *Yiyao lun*). This was followed by the denunciation of Chinese medicine and endless praise for Western medicine. Many famous people of the late Qing and Republican periods, such as Yan Fu (严复 1854–1921), Liang Qichao (梁启超 1873–1929), Chen Duxiu (陈独秀 1879–1942), Lu Xun (鲁迅 1881–1936), Hu Shi (胡适 1891–1962), and others, can all be considered extreme opponents of Chinese medicine. But the strange thing is, from the late Qing onward, no matter how often Chinese medicine suffered repeated attempts to stifle it, whether from government pressure, the influence of famous people, or the opposition of part of the masses, it would not wither away. Looking carefully into the reason for this, it is actually quite simple and can be stated in one sentence: Chinese medicine is clinically effective. Chinese medicine relies on its own strength! Observing the history of the late Qing and Republican eras with the documents of contemporary journals from the standpoint of the present, it is worth noting that there is something much greater than merely the history of medicine behind the violent, pulsing social zeitgeist that shaped the struggle and resistance of Chinese medicine. In China—an ancient civilization—there are two types of philosophical, cultural, and social worldviews undergoing a process of blending and evolving. In this process is a remarkable view into the history of social thought, and from it one can see the big picture from one detail (Translator's note: literally, "see a spot and recognize a leopard" [可从中窥 斑 见豹 ke congzhong kuiban jianbao]).

As scientific knowledge advances, usually one can distinguish quite quickly whether a particular technology is to be preserved or abandoned. But rarely in the history of global science is there a technology like ancient Chinese medicine that provokes love on one hand while inciting enmity and endless controversy on the other. Today we can look back to see many historical examples of the emergence of conflicts in late Qing and Republican journals, but also the many improved and public medical prescriptions that are linked to the development of today's Traditional Chinese Medicine. Contemporary Chinese researchers should not stop merely at writing history with an objective narrative; rather, they should dare to write analyses, draw conclusions, and make comparisons of science as a reflection for future knowledge. Today, perhaps more than ever, it is worth researching the differences between Traditional Chinese Medicine and Western medicine from a more macroscopic, more scientific perspective in order to situate the development of Chinese medicine and its future. At the publishing symposium, comrade Han Qide pointed out that Western medicine uses more statistical methods in researching the overall nature of the use of medical prescriptions, whereas Chinese medicine is directed toward each variegated individual, starting from a dialectical perspective of the balance of yin-yang and paying attention to each individual's particular characteristics. I think this kind of basic discrepancy in the development of contemporary science will increasingly emphasize the qualitative medical value of Chinese medicine vis-à-vis the quantitative focus of Western medicine, and will increasingly receive the attention and affirmation of the global medical world.

3   Humanist Reflections on Late Qing and Republican Chinese
       Medical Journals

Some scholars have raised the matter that both the Chinese and Western scholarly terminologies in early journals were translated quite coarsely, but the praiseworthy aspect is that each article has its own naturalistic thought and language, and most of them are not long and are thus very readable. Since the writing style is unique, the perspective is distinct, and they say exactly what they want to say, these articles provide a valuable and enormous archive of source material for scholars.

      The first journal that *The Compilation* incorporated is *Report of the Academy of Beneficial Aid*, which has been accepted by scholars as China's first medical school journal; from this type of precious periodical, we can see many very interesting topics of conversation. For example, this journal's section called "Medical History Answers" (医历答问 Yili dawen) follows the saying, "five movements and six qi[1] all begin in the Great Cold" (五运六气皆始于

---

1   This translation is from Nigel Wiseman, *Dictionary of Chinese Medicine, English-Chinese, Chinese-English* (Changsha: Hunan Science & Technology Press, 2006), 685, who offers the unorthodox alternate translation of the full term as "cosmobiology"; compare Shuai Xiezhong, *Changyong zhongyi mingci shuyu* (Terminology of traditional Chinese medicine) (Changsha: Hunan Science & Technology Press, 2005), 16: "five movements and six climates," explained as "The ancients combined the Theory of the Five Elements with the changes of the six kinds of climate (wind, heat, warmth, dampness, dryness, and chills) to deduce the relationship between the changes of weather and the occurrence of disease in humans. This

大寒 Wu yun liu qi jie shi yu Dahan) taking the lunar calendar "Great Cold" (大寒 Dahan) to the next year's "Little Cold" (小寒 Xiaohan) as comprising a full year from start to finish. In addition, it used a method of calculating time based on 15-day periods that was coordinated to methods of reckoning linked to the cycles of the human body in Chinese medicine taken from the *Basic Questions*' "Treatise on the Governance of the Five Constants" (素问五常政大论? Su wen—Wuchang zheng da lun), rather than the orthodox imperial calendar system. Some researchers claim this is merely an unorthodox alteration of the calendar, but it is more than that. Because imperial power was tied to calendric production, this innovation actually either displays a challenge to imperial power or shows that imperial power itself was weakening, because under normal circumstances the common people could not randomly change the imperially approved calendar at will.

Chinese medical journals frequently used the periodical form to advance distance education, and early on in correspondence education the student was called the "remote disciple" (遥从弟子 yao cong dizi). This type of educational method can be seen in the nineteenth century in England. When did China start having correspondence education? According to the *Cihai* dictionary's "correspondence education" entry, "China's first correspondence education organization was the correspondence school established by the Commercial Press in 1914." But looking at Chinese medical journals, we discover that the first correspondence school of Chinese medicine was actually established by Ding Fubao in his *Chinese-Western Medical Journal*. This journal was established in year two of the Qing Xuantong period (1910) in April; in the first issue is an advertisement seeking students for the New Medicine Lecture Society Correspondence School (刊发函授 新医学讲习社 Kan fa hanshou xin yixue jiangxi she), and it includes the general regulations for prospective students and a list of lectures, and so on. The regulations of the lecture society stipulate the study period as one year, with a test at the end of communications, and that those qualified would be given a certificate. Students would be charged a tuition of 2 dollars (*yuan*) per month, 70 cents (7 *jiao*) for teaching materials, and 30 cents (3 *jiao*) for postage. Those from poor families would have their fees reduced by half. The New Medicine Lecture Society Correspondence School established by the polymath Ding Fubao was aided by the *Chinese-Western Medical Journal* to maintain contact with remote disciples and trained a cohort of Chinese medical talent. For example, famous medical historian Chen Bangxian (陈邦贤 1889–1976) graduated from this school, receiving a certificate of

---

theory is somewhat similar to the modern climatological medicine and worthy of further investigation.

great distinction. The New Medicine Lecture Society Correspondence School started four years earlier than the Commercial Press Correspondence School, establishing itself as the forerunner of correspondence education in China, so researchers of educational history can obtain detailed information about early correspondence education in this journal. Speaking of education, the first issue of the *Report of the Academy of Beneficial Aid* had a section called "Beneficial Aid Medical Classics" (利济教经 Liji jiaojing) in the rhyming couplet format of the *Three Character Classic*, expressing its scope as including "rules and regulations of Chinese and Western studies, up to and including all of the world's activities." The content included traditional Chinese cultural knowledge, but also Western politics, culture, science, and technology, which Xiong Yuezhi has judged to be "the earliest self-compiled textbook of modern Chinese intellectuals," of great value for researching late Qing and Republican educational history.[2]

Aside from specializing in the particularities of Chinese medical periodicals, *The Compilation* also pays close attention to the establishment of special columns recording various kinds of medical news, medical terminology, random jottings, anecdotes, and other small stories, poems, and songs, and so on, which should all attract readers. This kind of content is very important information for researching Chinese medical culture, but is also a part of the research of late Qing and Republican society and literature. For example, *Shaoxing Medical Journal* has a column titled "Random Writings," which solicited local medical customs. General editor Qiu Jisheng's self-selected "Medical Customs of Shaoxing" introduces personal/family medicine, supernatural medicine, medicine of the rivers and lakes, official medicine, and semi-official medicine, treating the advance of popular vulgarizations and superstitions with sharp criticism. This information from a century ago is valuable material that would be difficult to otherwise obtain for those of us today who are researching local customs and regional culture. Moreover, this journal also carried humorous essays, rumors of the medical world, short stories, satire of contemporary problems—all humorous and interesting.

Another example is the second volume of *Guide to National Medicine* (国医 导报 Guoyi daobao), which established a column of "Random Jottings" (杂俎 Za zu) that published in succession Wu Quji's (吴去疾 dates unknown) "The Unofficial History of Physicians" (医林外史 Yilin wai shi), Huang Laoyi's (黄劳 逸 dates unknown) "Dreams and Human Life" (梦与人生 Meng yu rensheng) and "Alcohol and Human Life" (酒与人生 Jiu yu rensheng), Wang Yinghao's

---

2 Xiong Yuezhi, *The Dissemination of Western Learning and the Late Qing Society* (Shanghai Renmin chubanshe, 1994).

(王英豪 dates unknown) "Anecdotes of Medicine" (医林轶闻 Yilin yiwen), and others. *Guanghua Medical Magazine* (光华医药杂志 *Guanghua yiyao zazhi*) established columns such as "Interesting Research Information" (有趣的研究资料 Youqu de yanjiu ziliao), "Winter Silk Embroidery" (零缣寸锦 Ling jian cun jin), "Medical Literature and Art" (医林文艺 Yilin wenyi), and "Random Writings of the Artists" (艺林杂记 Yilin zaji). The *Shenzhou Medical Report* (神州医药学报 *Shenzhou yiyaoxue bao*) had columns for "Short Stories" (小说 Xiaoshuo) and "The Literary World" (文苑 Wenyuan); the first 30 issues collected a total of 12 short stories, among them Lian Xin's (莲心 dates unknown) social short story, "Perceptive" (燃犀 Ran xi), which was serialized in nine issues. The literature in journals of Chinese medicine was rather special. The content all had a connection with medicine, so it could perhaps be called "medical literature." In the process of editing, I also read a piece of writing attributed to Bing Xin (冰心 1900–1999), "Interesting Discussions on Medicine" (医药趣话 Yiyao qu hua), in *Annals of the Medical World* (医界春秋 *Yijie chunqiu*), issue nine. The writing style does not seem like that of Bing Xin's other works, but Bing Xin actually studied Western medicine for two years. I have not researched Bing Xin, but I believe that those scholars that do will be interested in reading it.

4   Correcting and Restoring History

Faced with such a rich cultural repository, having completed editing *The Compilation*, the collective desire of the editor and editorial team is to reduce any legacy of regrets as far as possible, but the compilation and editing of large-scale collectanea is inevitably a troublesome and difficult process. After the initial selection process, we discovered that almost no single library had complete runs of journals; in the process of supplementing collections, we also discovered that journals of this special subject were in terrible condition and it was rare for most large libraries to hold even one out of ten. Taking Shanghai Library as an example, this repository's collection is very rich and the collection on late Qing and Republican Chinese medical journals is among the best from all provincial and municipal libraries, but, of the 49 journals and more than 120,000 pages of material we collected in total, the collection at Shanghai Library only had about 10,000 pages. In order to make up the deficiency of pages, we investigated 50 libraries in succession, even contacting private collectors and the website "Confucius Old Books Network" (kongfz.com). We took no account of the cost of our networking, so that we would not regret missing unrecognized talent. If there was truly no way to supplement missing issues and pages missing from issues, we give an explanation, hoping that in the future there will be new discoveries. In the process of attempting to supplement incomplete runs, we discovered that many journals had experienced the ravages of time: pages had become brittle and weathered, and could not stand to be turned over for examination. Passing through the process of collation, printing, and publishing can cause these to be preserved, so the documents of the few can become many, transmitted to future generations, and we are secretly satisfied and feel gratified.

The Compilation reflects more than half a century of the development of Chinese medical history in the late Qing and Republican periods, yet also reveals more than half a century of social development history, with rich content; therefore those scholars at the publishing symposium for *The Compilation* regarded it as an "encyclopedia" of late Qing and Republican China. In order to maintain the long-term historical value of this "encyclopedia," in the editorial process we took preserving authenticity as the first priority, taking care with many tiny, insignificant details from the original publications. For example, in the early issues of *Report of the Academy of Beneficial Aid*, from issue 17 on we could not find the original journal, but Wenzhou Library had a notebook in which the content of the original journal had been compiled in sections. In the process of editing, according to the original journal form we compiled it as an "addendum" to preserve its authenticity. Another example was *Medical News*, which was also like this—the original classic was cropped and bound so that it was difficult to see the true nature of the original. In the process of editing, we reattached the content pieces together, for the convenience of the reader. Moreover, something worth paying attention to is the journals' advertisements. These advertisements include introductions to practicing physicians, publicity for Chinese-Western pharmaceutical patent medicines, and news of medical publications, and so on, by no means isolated cases, so that they could provide a multifaceted use for researching industrial, pharmaceutical, and medical book culture. We even went so far as to take some pages that had been interposed in the journals, such as reader contact cards, reader opinion solicitation forms, and purchase order requests, to make appendices that we printed after that issue of the journal, even to the point of reproducing a single page with a single word—all was precious and we wanted to satisfy the needs of many different researchers.

Senior document scholar Deng Jinsheng (郑金生 1946-), the former head of the Documents Research Committee of the Institute of Chinese Medical Science, has already expended enormous effort in researching late Qing and Republican Chinese medical journals, and is fully aware that acquiring extant copies is not easy due to their being scattered all over the country. At *The*

Compilation publishing symposium, Deng spoke to us, demonstrating his deep gratification at being able to see the successful completion of such a collection. While researching one kind of journal, he had been able to advise quite a few Ph.D. students, but with the publication of this large collection he could advise even more! To see him so deeply moved made me think of my participation in last year's editorial board working conference on the fifth compilation of the *Republican Collectanea* (民国丛书 *Minguo congshu*)—scholars said that it was the publication of the *Republican Collectanea* that promoted research of Republican scholarly history. This is not a bad saying—if there had been no *Republican Collectanea*, then many original texts would be hard to find, and researching Republican scholarship would be easier said than done. I also hope that the publication of *The Compilation* will likewise promote vigorous historical scholarship on late Qing and Republican Chinese medicine and related humanities research.

After all of the edited books were published, the editorial committee immediately started editing and publishing work on two reference works for this collection: an abstracted table of contents (中国近代中医药期刊汇编总目提要 *Zhongguo jindai zhongyiyao qikan huibian zongmu tiyao*) and an index (中国近代中医药期刊汇编索引 *Zhongguo jindai zhongyiyao qikan huibian suoyin*). Currently, the *Abstracted Table of Contents* has already been published, while work on the *Index* has been intensified and it will be published by the end of 2014. I believe that the publication of this set of two accompanying reference works will facilitate even more scholarly use of this large-scale collection.

Printed in the United States
By Bookmasters